YOUR
PREGNANCY
MD

the **FIRST** trimester

Dr. James W. Brann

ISBN 978-1450575959

Designed by Ashley McPeak
Edited by Doan Phuong Nguyen

Our mission is to guide you through your pregnancy with helpful and beneficial information.
We are committed to providing information that relates to all types of women, not any one
individual person's health. Be aware that the information we provide may or may not relate to
your particular situation. You should always consult your doctor or health care professional
before acting on any information you may read in this book.

The publisher, author(s) and owner are not offering medical advice. It is important that you
recognize you must rely on the advice of your medical professional for guidance regarding
your healthcare.

First Edition: March 2010

Website: WomensHealthCareTopics.com

{Contents}

Welcome to the Start of an Amazing Journey!

Letter from Dr. James Brann . . . .

Becoming a mother is one of the most exhilarating times in any woman's life. Pregnancy is a special time, despite the uncomfortable symptoms and physical changes that it brings. As you feel another life growing within you, needing you for his or her nutrition and support, you will feel an immense, unconditional love that cannot be matched. It's often said that pregnant women are more beautiful and have a special glow about them. Not only is this due to the love that you have for your little baby, but it's also the excitement that you feel as you await your little one's arrival into the world.

Pregnancy is broken up into three trimesters. While each is equally important, this book focuses only on the first trimester of pregnancy—the first 13 weeks. This is a critical time in your baby's development as his or her brain, spinal cord, nervous system, heart, and other organs are forming. Anything that you do and consume (such as smoking, drinking, and drugs) can hurt your baby, more severely in the first trimester than later in the pregnancy.

If you think of pregnancy as a continuum, each part on the pregnancy timeline comes with its own set of problems. This book presents everything you will need to know about early pregnancy—symptoms you may experience, changes to expect, and pregnancy complications that may occur.

As a retired obstetrician with 26 years of experience, I have witnessed the miracle of life thousands of times. I know first hand the concerns and questions that expectant mothers have. I hope to address many of these issues in this book. I aim to offer you the same level of expertise that I offer my patients to alleviate any concerns you may have about the first trimester of your pregnancy.

Best Wishes,

James Brann m.o.

THE LENGTH OF PREGNANCY EXPLAINED

You may be asking yourself, "Why does this book start off with week 4? What about weeks 1, 2, and 3?"

Although the day of conception is literally when you first became pregnant, doctors don't think that way. It's too imprecise. There is no surefire way of knowing which day you actually ovulated and conceived, because there are many variables that come into play to complicate ovulation.

Doctors calculate the start of your pregnancy with the first day of your last menstrual period. Most women do not know their estimated day of conception, but they can often pinpoint the date of their last period. Therefore, it is easier for healthcare professionals and doctors to use your period to calculate pregnancy.

A regular menstrual cycle is 28 days, and most women ovulate around 2 weeks (or 14 days) after their period begins. So your estimated date of conception is likely two weeks after your period.

Because you may not know that you are pregnant until week 4, when you realize your period has not returned, week 4 is the perfect place to start this book!

We have divided pregnancy into weeks. Counting weeks is more precise than months, as there will always be 7 days in a week. The number of days and weeks in a month fluctuates, making it less precise.

The weeks of pregnancy are divided into three trimesters. Each trimester lasts about 13 to 14 weeks, or about 3 months.

- 1st trimester: 0-13 weeks
- 2nd trimester: 14-28 weeks
- 3rd trimester: 29-40 weeks

A normal pregnancy lasts between 37 to 42 weeks. Babies born before 37 weeks are considered "preterm," and a pregnancy that lasts more than 42 weeks is considered "post-term."

{**Fun Fact**} You can calculate your estimated due date by using Naegle's Rule. Simply subtract three months from the date of your last menstrual period and add seven days. So if your last period was February 20th, then you will deliver your baby on November 27th. This rule assumes that you have a regular 28-day menstrual cycle with conception occurring on day 14.

HOW THIS BOOK IS ORGANIZED

Your Pregnancy MD: The First Trimester guides you through every week of your first trimester, starting with week 4—the week that most women first realize they are pregnant.

Every chapter is broken into five sections (except for weeks 4, 8, and 12, which have a bonus prenatal care section!):

Fetal Development

Track your baby's development week-by-week. You will be amazed at how much your little one grows. The first trimester is a critical time in your baby's development as all his major organs are developing. Your risk of miscarriage is much higher in the first trimester than at any other time of pregnancy.

Mom's Pregnancy Symptoms

With the significant changes that your little one is undergoing, it's no wonder your pregnancy hormones are going crazy! You will feel those uncomfortable pregnancy symptoms almost immediately. From morning sickness to breast tenderness, the first trimester of pregnancy is not always glamorous.

Pregnancy 411

In this section, we discuss need-to-know information that relates to your first trimester of pregnancy, including lifestyle choices and how they may affect your pregnancy, health and nutrition issues, prenatal tests, how to take care of yourself during these critical weeks, and much more.

Normal Changes to Expect

This section covers in-depth changes that you should expect to experience in your first trimester. These changes are not always pleasant, but we provide helpful tips and fun facts to help you cope.

Complications During Pregnancy

Although every woman hopes to have a smooth and easy pregnancy, complications can occur. Learn about specific complications that can arise during the first trimester of pregnancy, including how certain illnesses can create problems for your baby.

Prenatal Care

A bonus section on the weeks that you will be visiting your doctor, this section prepares you for your prenatal care visits and highlights what you should expect.

WEEK 4

Could you be pregnant?
What does this all mean?

Letter from Dr. James Brann

It's been four weeks since your last period, and you're experiencing a few pregnancy symptoms, such as morning sickness and fatigue, but no signs of a period. Could you be pregnant? What does this all mean?

Run to your nearest drugstore for a pregnancy test to find out. If the test is positive, notify your physician to take a pregnancy test from their office.

If you are indeed pregnant, congratulations! The road to parenthood is an exciting journey filled with many ups and downs. Over the next 40 weeks, your body is undergoing some amazing changes as your bundle of joy grows within you.

At this very early stage of pregnancy, you will be in awe to learn what's happening inside your womb at this very moment! It's been two weeks since conception, and your new life is no longer just a ball of cells. In the next few weeks, he or she is hurling toward looking more and more like a tiny human being!

Best Wishes,

James Brann m.d.

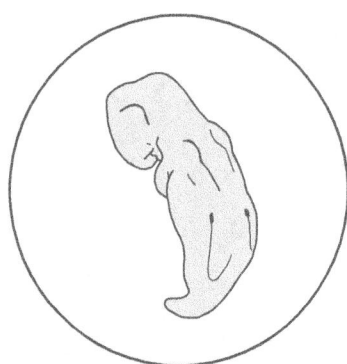

FETAL DEVELOPMENT

Within twenty-four hours of conception, after your partner's sperm has fertilized your egg, the egg begins dividing into many cells. In that first week, your soon-to-be baby is just a tiny ball of cells that moves through your fallopian tube into the uterus, where it implants itself and begins to grow.

Most women discover they are pregnant at 4 weeks. By this time, two weeks have passed since conception. Your baby is quickly changing into something that resembles a tiny tadpole. In less than 36 weeks, he or she may be a 7 pound baby!

At week 4, your baby is still incredibly miniscule! It is only about .014 to .04 inches long, which is about 1/2 to 1 mm long.

Your baby's development is still in its earliest stages. Your little one is working furiously to embed itself deeper and deeper into the lining of your uterus to ensure a safe home for the next 9 months.

The life-support system of your baby – called the placenta – is developing this week. The placenta will help nourish and support the baby throughout its development; it supplies oxygen and nutrients to the baby, and removes wastes. The waste is returned to your blood stream so that your kidneys can get rid of it. The umbilical cord connects the placenta to the baby.

By this week, two cell layers have formed. One of these layers will form the baby's "yolk sac," which provides nutrients to the tiny baby early in its development. The other layer will eventually form the body of your child.

{**Fact**} A delay in the reading of your pregnancy test can give you a false positive, so be sure and follow the directions accurately!

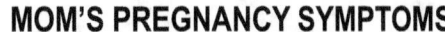

MOM'S PREGNANCY SYMPTOMS

Week 4 is often the time when women begin to wonder if they are pregnant or not. Many women notice a missed period – which may signal that conception (fertilization of the egg) and implantation (the embryo attaching to the uterus) has taken place.

With the advances in testing technology, over-the-counter pregnancy tests can be accurate as early as the first day of a missed period. These pregnancy kits measure the pregnancy hormone hCG (human Chorionic Gonadotropin) in your urine. However, a pregnancy test at your doctor's office is always a surefire way to find out if you are pregnanct or not.

> **{Tip}** If you initially test negative but your period still doesn't start when it should, wait a day or two and take another pregnancy test. As more time passes, the test results will become more reliable.

Although some women may not get their period again until after the baby comes, others may experience slight spotting or brownish staining early in their pregnancy. Spotting can occur six to eight days after fertilization. As the fertilized egg is burrowing itself into the lining of your uterus, it can cause you to experience a small amount of blood, called "implantation bleeding." Don't confuse this spotting with menstrual bleeding, which tends to be heavier and for a longer period of time.

During this week, you may also begin to experience some early pregnancy symptoms. The most common include nausea with or without vomiting, breast tenderness, fatigue, and an increased need to urinate.

> **{Fact}** Vaginal bleeding early in pregnancy does not necessarily mean that anything is wrong. Check with your physician to make sure.

PREGNANCY 411

Early Pregnancy Changes

By the time many women have realized that they have missed their period, they have already begun to experience some early symptoms of pregnancy. These may include:

• **Nausea and vomiting** - Also called "morning sickness," this is a common complaint of pregnancy. You may start to feel nauseous right away. Some women experience nausea and vomiting together. Either way, it is not a pleasant experience. Luckily, morning sickness tends to go away in the second trimester.

• **Breast sensitivity and enlargement** - When you're pregnant, your breasts may become tender, tingle, swell, and feel sore or very sensitive to touch.

• **Overall Fatigue** - An almost universal pregnant symptom in early pregnancy is fatigue. You tire easily and need more rest.

• **Feeling Bloated** - This bloating sensation is similar to what you may have experienced during your regular menstrual cycle.

• **Urinary Frequency** - You might have the need to urinate more often as soon as you become pregnant. This is a common pregnancy symptom that can become a nuisance.

• **Lack of Energy** - As your body adjusts to the increasing pregnancy hormones, your energy level will take a hit. Your energy tends to be lower than before pregnancy.

Overview of Lifestyle Choices

Now that you think you might be pregnant, you need to start examining your health and lifestyle choices. A healthy lifestyle is key for a successful pregnancy. The choices you make now in your daily life can affect both your health and the health of your unborn child.

You should avoid bad habits when you are pregnant. These include smoking, drinking, and using drugs. Not only do these habits expose your baby to harmful chemicals that can be detrimental to his/her health and development, they can also affect your overall health and well-being.

Smoking during pregnancy can increase the risk of an ectopic pregnancy, vaginal bleeding, stillbirths (delivering a baby with no heartbeat), and delivering a low-birth-weight baby.

Drinking any alcohol during pregnancy is not recommended. Chronic alcohol abuse early in pregnancy can lead to fetal alcohol syndrome, an increased risk of a miscarriage, and delivering a premature baby.

Abusing drugs during pregnancy is extremely detrimental to your baby. It can lead to long-term health problems, and your baby may need special care after birth. During pregnancy, drug use can stunt fetal growth as well as brain growth. You are also at an increased risk of delivering a premature baby.

In addition to avoiding bad habits, remember to eat a balanced and healthy diet. We will discuss this in more detail in future chapters, but maintaining a healthy diet will give your little one the nutrients and vitamins he/she needs to develop into a healthy baby.

Exercise also has many benefits during pregnancy. If you don't exercise regularly, now would be a great time to start. Not only will exercise prep your body for labor and delivery, it can increase your energy level; relieve constipation, bloating, swelling, and leg cramps; help you relax and feel better; improve your sleep; and control gestational diabetes.

> **{Tip}** Ideas for safe exercises include walking, swimming, cycling, jogging, aerobics, yoga, Pilates, golf, bowling, and strength training. Be sure to avoid any sports that may increase your risk of falling—like racquet sports, horseback riding, downhill snow skiing, and contact sports.

As with any kind of exercise program, be sure to discuss your plans with your doctor.

NORMAL CHANGES TO EXPECT

Early Breast Changes

Swollen and tender breasts are often the first clue that many women have that they may be pregnant. Throughout your pregnancy, expect that your breasts will get bigger in size and heavier in weight, as the fat layer of your breasts thickens and the number of milk glands increases.

You may notice that as your breasts are becoming heavier, they start to tingle and feel sore. Some women also experience sensitivity to touch. At first, the sensations will be similar to the swollen breasts that you get just prior to your menstrual cycle. As your pregnancy progresses, they will increase in tenderness.

A good maternity bra may help relieve some of your tenderness. These bras are manufactured with wider straps, larger cups to protect your growing breasts, and extra hooks to adjust the band size, as your breasts grows bigger. You might also want to buy a special sleep bra for support during the night.

{**Fun Fact**} Because the early signs of pregnancy, including tender breasts, are similar to common PMS (premenstrual syndrome) symptoms, women with irregular periods may not realize they are pregnant until much later.

Early Pregnancy Spotting

You have all the classic signs of pregnancy, but you're experiencing light vaginal spotting. It looks like a very light period—you may have one or two spots of bright red blood, or it may be coffee ground in appearance. But you have no cramping or pain accompanying this bleeding. What's going on?

Don't worry! This light bleeding, called "spotting" or "staining," is a very common occurrence in early pregnancy. Between 20 and 40 percent of pregnant women experience vaginal spotting in their first trimester. The major reasons why spotting occurs includes a possible miscarriage, implantation bleeding, and ectopic pregnancies.

In more than 50 percent of the women who bleed early in their pregnancies, the bleeding stops as their pregnancy progresses. However, in some unfortunate cases, women may experience heavy bleeding, accompanied with painful cramps, and this can end in a miscarriage.

Because spotting looks very similar to a light period, some pregnant women do confuse this phenomenon with having a menstrual period. If the over-the-counter pregnancy test comes back positive and you're experiencing spotting, you should seek medical help immediately to find out what's going on.

{Fact} You may experience spotting and light bleeding immediately after sexual intercourse. Hormonal changes during pregnancy causes the surface of your cervix to become more fragile and "raw," which can cause bleeding.

COMPLICATIONS DURING PREGNANCY

Ectopic Tubal Pregnancy

Although many women with spotting in the first trimester continue on to term without any major complications, spotting that comes with cramps or severe abdominal pain can be a sign of a miscarriage or an ectopic pregnancy.

An ectopic pregnancy can also have virtually no symptoms, which is why scheduling your first prenatal visit is essential to the health of you and your baby.

In a regular pregnancy, your fertilized egg travels through one of your fallopian tubes to the lining of your uterus, where it embeds itself and starts to grow. In an ectopic pregnancy, the fertilized egg embeds itself in a location outside your uterus. About 98 percent of all ectopic pregnancies occur within one of your fallopian tubes. When this happens, it is called a "tubal pregnancy." In rare cases, ectopic pregnancies can occur in an ovary, cervix, or abdomen.

Tubal pregnancies are often caused by damage to the fallopian tubes. This damage may be scarring of the tube, as a result of past ectopic pregnancies, past tubal infections, or surgery to the tube. This scarring can block or slow the movement of the fertilized egg as it travels from the fallopian tube to the uterus.

{**Fact**} Up to half of the women who have ectopic pregnancies have pelvic inflammatory disease or swelling of their fallopian tubes.

Because space is limited in the fallopian tubes, the baby does not have the room to grow and the pregnancy cannot develop as it should and must be treated.

If an ectopic pregnancy in a fallopian tube is allowed to grow inside your fallopian tube, the tube can rupture, causing major internal bleeding in the mother. This can become life threatening. In this extreme case, the ectopic pregnancy is treated with surgery. The ruptured tube may have to be removed, which means the woman has to rely on her remaining fallopian tube for future pregnancies.

More than 50 percent of women with ectopic pregnancies have no symptoms until their fallopian tube ruptures. After the tube ruptures, women may experience severe pain and heavy vaginal bleeding. Dizziness, a lowering of blood pressure, fainting, and shock are also symptoms.

When ectopic pregnancies are caught early and the tube has not ruptured, it can be treated medically or surgically.

Sometimes, an ectopic pregnancy in the fallopian tube resolves on its own. Called "tubal abortion" this occurs when the embryo is expelled from the fallopian tube before it ruptures. The woman who experiences tubal abortions may have severe vaginal bleeding that requires surgery or have minimal bleeding that doesn't require any medical treatment.

The good news: around 89 percent of women with previous ectopic pregnancies can go on to have regular pregnancies and deliver babies to term. Ectopic pregnancies are diagnosed with transvaginal ultrasounds and a special blood test that measures the pregnancy hormone, hCG (human Chorionic Gonadotropin).

{**Fact**} **One in 50 pregnancies is ectopic. Ectopic pregnancies have become more common within the last several decades. Women who have had a previous ectopic pregnancy have a 15 percent chance of having another.**

Any woman of childbearing age can be at risk for an ectopic pregnancy, but those with abnormal fallopian tubes are at higher risk. These include women with a history of pelvic inflammatory disease, previous ectopic pregnancies, infertility, pelvic or abdominal surgery, endometriosis (a condition in which the tissue that lines your uterus grows outside the womb), sexually transmitted disease, and prior tubal surgery (like tubal sterilization). The morning after pill has also been linked to some cases of ectopic pregnancies.

Older women (over 35), smokers, and women who have been exposed to the drug diethylstilbestrol (DES) during her mother's pregnancy are at an even higher risk for an ectopic pregnancy.

PRENATAL CARE

Choosing the Right Doctor

As soon as you become pregnant, you will want to find a good doctor to take care of you and your baby for the next nine months. But how do you go about doing this?

First, interview friends, relatives, and medical professionals. Ask anyone whose opinion you trust. Find out which doctors they liked, which they didn't, and ask why. Then, ask yourself whether you are more comfortable with a male or female doctor. Think about what hospital you want to deliver your baby at, and if you want a doctor or midwife. Do you want a sole practitioner or a doctor from a large practice?

A sole practitioner gives you personal care. They will know all about you and your needs, but they may not be available when you deliver. This may put you in the hands of an unfamiliar doctor.

On the other hand, a doctor who is part of a large practice or medical group may offer you an impersonal experience, but you will see most of the doctors at least once, so if your preferred doctor is unavailable for your delivery, you will still be working with a doctor that you've already met.

When interviewing a potential physician, here are a few questions you may want to ask:

- Are you affiliated with the American College of Obstetrics and Gynecology? Are you board certified?

- How many years have you been in practice?

- Are there nurse practitioners, midwives, or physician assistants in the practice? What roles do they play in patient care?

- Do you have a vacation scheduled that coincides with my due date?

- How many babies have you delivered? What percentage was vaginal? Cesarean? Induced?

- What is your position on pain control?

- Do you support the use of doulas (professional labor coaches who provide physical and emotional support during labor and birth)?

• Do you support a particular birthing technique? (Lamaze and Bradley are the most common)

{**Fun Fact**} The Lamaze technique and the Bradley method are common childbirth classes that promote breathing, relaxation, and exercise during labor and delivery. Lamaze, the most popular method in the U.S., encourages the mother to deal with pain through training and preparation (called psychoprophylaxis). The Bradley method (also called "husband-coached birth") emphasizes a natural birth with the avoidance of medications unless absolutely necessary. Bradley is often the preferred method for women who want to give birth at home or in a nonhospital setting.

• Does your practice offer breastfeeding support?

• In an emergency situation or in the case that you are unavailable for labor and delivery, who will serve as your backup?

• Do you support the use of birth plans (a written outline defining your delivery care – what you want to happen during labor and delivery, the setting you want to deliver in, the pain medications you want to use, and etc.)?

• How are questions and concerns you may have between visits handled?

Once you have decided on that special doctor, call and schedule your first prenatal appointment. Call right away, because it may be a few weeks before you see the doctor.

For the first 28 weeks of pregnancy, you will generally have prenatal visits every 4 weeks. Then, between 28 and 36 weeks, you will see the doctor every 2 weeks. After 36 weeks until you deliver, you will have appointments every week. Women who have medical problems, as well as teenagers, may require more frequent appointments. Your doctor will set up the appropriate intervals for your scheduled visits, depending on the nature and severity of any problems that may arise.

WEEK

5

The week of the "wow" shock factor

Letter from Dr. James Brann · · · · · · · · · · · · · · · · ·

In my practice, this is the week that has more of a "wow" shock factor than any other time during pregnancy. By week 5, more pregnancy symptoms have begun to appear and the reality of pregnancy is finally sinking in.

This is an emotional time for my patients as they feel anguish over the thought of starting a family and the responsibilities that come with it. Others may experience pure excitement and elation, but worry about the health and safety of their growing baby.

It is very common at this early stage of pregnancy for women to come into their doctor's office with spotting (light bleeding during pregnancy that looks similar to period blood), full of worry about miscarriage. In a majority of cases, spotting is nothing to worry about and may be due to implantation bleeding—which happens when the fertilized egg attaches to the uterus.

In rare cases, vaginal bleeding in the first trimester may be a sign of molar pregnancy (which I have explained in detail under the "Complications During Pregnancy" section in this chapter).

Your baby is undergoing important changes this week – including the formation of his or her heart!

Best Wishes,

James Brann m.d.

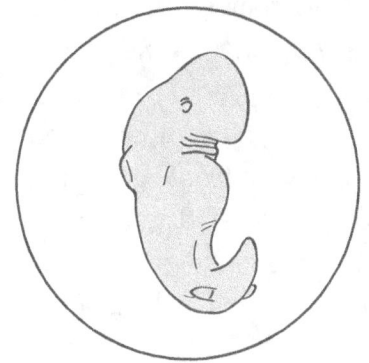

FETAL DEVELOPMENT

This week is very similar to week 4. Your baby is still extremely tiny and measures at just over a millimeter long. Vital organs are continuing to grow and develop this week and big changes are underway.

By week 5, your baby's brain is dividing into three primary sections: the "forebrain," "midbrain," and "hindbrain." The forebrain will eventually control the baby's movement, memory, emotions, thinking, and speech. The midbrain plays a role in your little one's vision, hearing, eye and body movement. The hindbrain controls balance and coordination.

{**Fun Fact**} **Your baby's umbilical cord, though still short, now connects him or her to the developing placenta.**

The respiratory and digestive systems are also developing this week. The primitive placenta and umbilical cord are forming.

As the first blood cells make their way into the yolk sac, blood vessels begin to form throughout your baby and the beginnings of a heart emerges. Separate chambers quickly begin to develop and start pumping blood.

During week 5, the tiny body of your baby is starting to form, as the brain, spinal cord, and heart have become identifiable alongside the yolk sac.

Because of its rapid growth, the relatively flat embryo begins to fold, incorporating part of the yolk sac into the lining of the digestive system. This process forms the chest and abdominal cavities of your tiny developing baby.

{**Fun Fact**} The circulatory system is the first group of related organs to achieve a functional state.

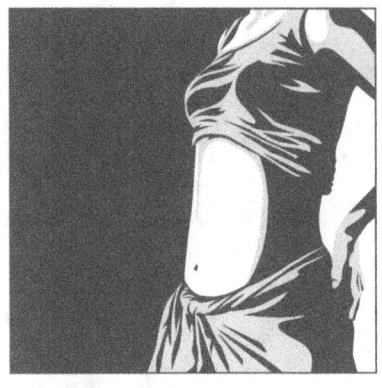

MOM'S PREGNANCY SYMPTOMS

Since your baby is extremely small, you won't be noticeably pregnant at week 5. Some women, especially mothers who have given birth before, have reported that they noticed feeling more bloating and that their lower abdomen was starting to pouch out. However, first-time mothers may not notice any significant abdominal changes for a few more weeks.

During these first early weeks of pregnancy, many women experience worry and concern over the health of their growing baby. Don't be too hard on yourself if you're going through these emotions—they are absolutely normal. Lean on loved ones and your partner, and talk about your feelings. Be sure to rest and relax, as this may make you feel better and calmer.

At week 5, you may experience some fatigue. Fatigue is common in the first trimester and less so in the second trimester. If your fatigue doesn't improve after week 12, it's possible that there is a secondary cause, which may include depression, stress, or lifestyle issues.

As the weeks pass by, you may experience the need to urinate more often. This is a common complaint for many pregnant women, and there are several reasons for this. First, doctors recommend that pregnant women drink more during pregnancy to keep hydrated. In addition, your kidneys are working extra hard to flush waste products out of your body. As your baby grows inside you and your uterus becomes larger, it puts more pressure on your bladder, making you feel like it's full. As a result, you'll make extra trips to the bathroom.

{Tip} Having too many urine leaks? Try Kegel exercises! These help strengthen the muscles that surround your urethra – the tube that carries urine out of the body. To do Kegel exercises, simple squeeze the muscles you use to stop peeing. Hold for 10 seconds, and then release.

PREGNANCY 411

Nutrition

When you're pregnant, proper nutrition and a balanced diet are essential to the health of you and your baby. The added nutritional demands that pregnancy places on your body requires you to start making good lifestyle choices—like choosing the right foods to eat and maintaining a healthy weight gain.

As the old saying goes, you are eating for two! Your diet should include a combination of proteins, carbohydrates, vitamins and minerals, and fat. These will fuel your body, make you feel better, and nourish your growing baby.

{Fun Fact} If you already have good eating habits, eating a proper balanced diet will take little effort; just add 300 extra calories to your normal diet.

Pregnancy also brings on food cravings in some women. Most often, giving into your cravings isn't harmful. It only causes problems when you eat too much of one thing and abandon the rest of your diet.

Check out the Food Guide Pyramid to help you maintain a balanced diet. It will guide you and show you the correct servings for each major food group. Although it's not designed for pregnancy, it gives you a good idea on the types of food you should eat. The food pyramid guide emphasizes diets that are low in fat, sugar and cholesterol, while high in fruits, vegetables and grains.

In addition to eating healthy food, many women should take prenatal vitamins to make sure that they get enough nutrients in their diet. Certain vitamins are very important for your baby's growth—such as folic acid, iron, and calcium.

Both iron and folic acid aid your body in making the extra blood your body needs to keep you and your baby healthy. Folic acid is probably one of the most important nutrients you need during pregnancy. It reduces your baby's risk of neural tube defects—birth defects that happen due to incomplete development of the spine—and it decreases your chances for vascular problems, like heart disease.

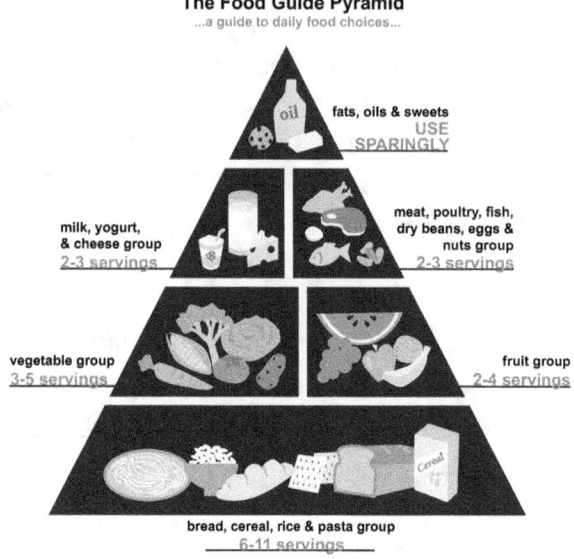

Calcium helps your baby develop stronger bones and teeth. If your body lacks enough calcium during pregnancy, your baby will rob the calcium from your bones—which will make them weak and brittle.

NORMAL CHANGES TO EXPECT

Fatigue

Many pregnant women report fatigue as one of their most wearisome symptoms. Like other pregnancy symptoms, your pregnancy hormones – especially the rising levels of progesterone – can contribute to your increased fatigue. In addition, your body is using a bulk of its energy to create and support the baby growing inside you.

Your fatigue tends to exhaust you during the first trimester, then gets better during the second trimester, and gets worse during the third trimester. In the third trimester, your energy level may drop due to the extra weight you're carrying, as your baby is getting larger.

To deal with your fatigue, you may want to go to bed earlier and try to get at least 8 hours of sleep; take a 15-minute nap every day; eat healthy mini meals instead of a large one; and exercise every day.

> {**Fact**} At the beginning of your second trimester, your energy level should be increasing. If your fatigue continues, you may have anemia or depression.

Fainting and Dizziness

Experiencing some dizziness or light-headedness when you are pregnant is a very common occurrence, and it should not cause you to worry too much.

Dizziness can occur when you stand up too quickly or stay standing for a long period of time, because all your blood flows to the lowest part of your body (to your legs) and not enough oxygen is available to your brain, causing you to experience light-headedness. Lying on your back can also cause you to become dizzy, because the weight of your uterus pushes on a huge vein, called the vena cava (which supplies blood from your legs to your heart), and cuts off the blood supply to your heart.

Although dizziness is normal during pregnancy, if you don't fix what's causing you to feel light-headed, you can faint.

If you start feeling faint, immediately lie down on your left side to increase the blood flow to your brain. You should feel better within a few minutes. Other ways to relieve this sensation include trying to keep cool, keeping hydrated with lots of water and fluids, avoid rising too quickly or getting out of bed too fast.

> {**Tip**} If you're feeling light-headed and you are driving a car, pull over immediately and shift your weight to your left hip.

COMPLICATIONS DURING PREGNANCY

Miscarriage Risk with Intrauterine Device (IUD)

The intrauterine device (IUD) is one of the oldest methods of contraception and is used worldwide by many women to prevent pregnancy. Like other birth control devices, it is not always 100 percent effective. Women can still conceive with an IUD in place. Your risk of pregnancy is the highest in the first year after you get the IUD inserted.

Unfortunately, women who get pregnant while using an IUD have a very high risk of a miscarriage—between 40 to 50 percent. Because of this increased risk, it is essential to remove the IUD as soon as possible. This will decrease the risk of losing the baby.

It is better to remove the IUD in the first trimester rather than waiting, as there will be fewer complications. Within the first trimester, if the IUD strings are visible, removal is easy. Sometimes, removal may not be possible if the IUD strings are not visible or if your doctors deem that removal of the IUD will be too difficult or will disrupt the safety of the pregnancy.

If the IUD remains in place after the second trimester, the woman has four times the risk of delivering a preterm baby. Removing the IUD at this point may also increase the risk of miscarriage, fetal trauma, and bleeding.

> **{Fact}** 15 to 20 percent of all pregnancies end in miscarriage. It normally occurs within the first three months of pregnancy.

Gestational Trophoblastic Disease (GTD) or Molar Pregnancies

Molar pregnancies – also known as gestational trophoblastic disease (GTD) – are a very rare but serious complication that can occur early in pregnancy. It occurs in one out of every 1,000 to 1,200 pregnancies.

Both normal and molar pregnancies develop as a result of a fertilized egg. But in a molar pregnancy, the fertilized egg doesn't grow into a healthy baby; instead, abnormal cells grow and form into a mass of cells. A molar pregnancy is basically a tumor that develops in your uterus, where a baby should be growing.

Two types of molar pregnancies exist: complete and partial.

In a complete molar pregnancy, the fertilized egg never develops into an embryo but it grows into a grapelike cluster of tissue. In a partial molar pregnancy, the placenta grows into the molar tissue (the tumor), and any fetus that develops will have severe defects and will die in the womb. In rare circumstances, a twin pregnancy has been found to have one normal, healthy baby and one complete mole twin.

Molar pregnancies are considered "accidents of nature" and no one's fault. They are not caused by lifestyle or behavior; however, they are more common in older mothers (over 35 years of age).

Signs that you may have a molar pregnancy include vaginal bleeding during your first trimester, the passing of tissue through your vagina, pelvic pressure or pain.

Most molar pregnancies are treated with surgery under general anesthesia. Follow-up visits to the doctor are extremely important. These are to ensure that the molar pregnancy has been completely removed from your body. If traces of the mole remain, they can grow into cancerous tumors that pose threat to other parts of your body. Another attempt at pregnancy should be avoided for at least a year after your molar pregnancy.

{Fact} A majority of molar pregnancies (up to 87 percent) would be girl babies.

WEEK

6

Lots of exciting changes are happening this week!

Letter from Dr. James Brann •

As you'll discover, lots of exciting changes are happening this week. It is extremely vital at this stage of your pregnancy that you review your lifestyle choices and change habits that could be harmful to the baby.

It is common knowledge that smoking, alcohol, and drug use during pregnancy can be dangerous to the baby, but did you know that your caffeine intake could also affect the little one growing inside you? Research has linked caffeine consumption to possibly increasing the risk of miscarriage. Learn more about what foods to avoid during pregnancy in the "Pregnancy 411" section of this chapter.

Week 6 is the week that many of my patients come in with concerns over morning sickness. Although this is a relatively universal pregnancy symptom, different techniques work for different women. Some of my patients find that eating small mini meals all day long helps. Others complain that their prenatal vitamins are making them nauseous. If you experience this, you may want to try taking your vitamins at night or switch to chewable multi-vitamins or gummy bear vitamins.

As you battle with morning sickness and other pregnancy symptoms, your baby is developing rapidly within you. His or her limbs and face are starting to take shape in week 6! How exciting is that?

Best Wishes,

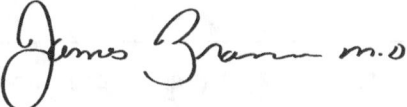

FETAL DEVELOPMENT

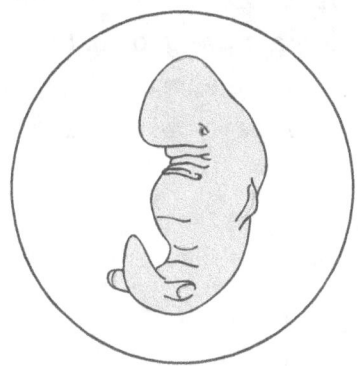

By week 6, your baby is finally big enough to be measured by an ultrasound. The measurements will be in increments referred to as "crown to rump length" – which is basically the top of your baby's head to the bottom of its buttocks. During this week, your obstetrician may also be able to see the baby's heartbeat, though it will not be until 12 weeks pregnant that a Doppler ultrasound (a small, hand-held device that is placed on your stomach) can detect the heartbeat. Ever so quickly, your baby is starting to look more and more like a tiny organic being!

At this early stage of development, your baby measures about 2 to 5 mm from crown to rump – about the size of a baby pea!

Your baby's heart started beating around 3 weeks and 1 day after conception, and by week 6, he/she is averaging 113 beats per minute. Throughout your baby's short lifetime, his/her tiny heart has beat a total of 1,139,040 times!

{**Fun Fact**} Did you know that the heart changes colors as blood enters and exits its chambers with each beat?

During week 6, a fluid-filled sac, called an amniotic sac, forms around your embryo. The liquid inside the sac is called amniotic fluid, and it will support and protect the baby from injury during its time inside your womb.

This week, your little Einstein's brain is growing very rapidly, which is noticeable by the change in appearance of his/her forebrain, midbrain, and hindbrain.

> **{Fun Fact}** **Primitive brainwaves have been recorded as early as 6 weeks and 2 days!**

Your baby's face is starting to take shape this week. Dark spots are forming on his/her face where his/her eyes and nostrils are going to be. Small pits have formed on the sides of his/her head where the ears are going to develop. Tiny buds should have also formed by now, which will eventually form into arms and legs.

At this point, your baby's skin is completely transparent as it is only one cell thick. The skin is slowly thickening.

MOM'S PREGNANCY SYMPTOMS

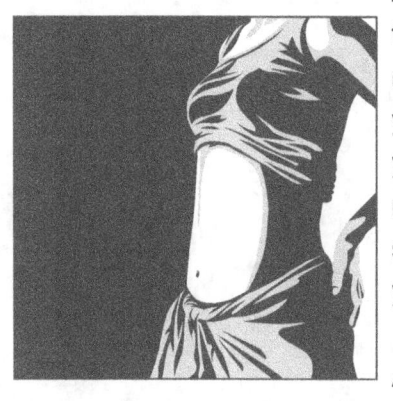

As your baby undergoes significant changes this week, you should expect to experience more subtle changes in your body. Although you probably haven't started to show yet, you'll definitely be feeling more pregnant by now. Be sure to get as much rest as possible in the upcoming weeks to help support your little one.

Are your pants getting tighter? Surprising as it may be, some women do experience weight gain this early on in their pregnancies. By week 6, most of the weight you gain is probably water weight. It's very common for women to start retaining fluid during pregnancy.

{**Fun Fact**} During your first trimester (up to week 12), it is very possible that you'll gain about five pounds.

Early in your pregnancy, you may notice that your breasts are swollen, tingling, or tender—similar sensations that you might experience before or during your menstrual cycle. Your breasts are continuing to grow to prepare for feeding your baby. By week 6, your breasts may have grown a whole bra-cup size. This may be due to several reasons: fat building up in your breasts and the number of milk glands increasing as your body is getting ready to produce milk for your little one.

Other breast changes that you might experience include a darkening of your nipples and areolas (the pink or brownish skin that surrounds your nipples), small bumps (called Montgomery's tubercles) on the surface of your areolas may start to form or become more pronounced than before, and more prominent veins may appear underneath your skin.

By now, you may have already experienced pregnancy-related nausea and vomiting – commonly known as morning sickness. This term is misleading, as morning sickness doesn't just happen in the morning; it can occur at any point during the day. This nausea just tends to be worse during the morning and can improve as the day continues.

PREGNANCY 411

Weight Gain in Pregnancy

In the last chapter, we learned how proper nutrition and a balanced diet can go a long way in maintaining the health of you and your growing baby. But did you know that your baby's birth weight is also affected by your pre-pregnancy weight and the weight you gain during pregnancy?

Fat babies may be super cute, but recent studies have shown that your baby's weight influences his/her future risk for developing diseases such as diabetes, high blood pressure, and heart disease.

Because your weight gain during your pregnancy is critical to you and your baby's health, it's important to understand how the weight you gain during pregnancy gets distributed in your body.

WHERE DOES THE WEIGHT GO?	
BABY	7 to 8 lbs
FAT	6 to 8 lbs
INCREASE IN BLOOD SUPPLY	3 to 4 lbs
WATER RETENTION	2 to 3 lbs
AMNIOTIC FLUID	2 lbs
BREAST ENLARGEMENT	3 lbs
UTERUS	2 lbs
AFTERBIRTH (PLACENTA)	1.5 lbs

For a happy outcome at the end of your pregnancy – a healthy baby – you have to be careful about your total weight gain. More than 50 percent of women gain either too much or too little during their pregnancy, and this can be harmful to your baby's safety.

Your starting weight determines your recommended pregnancy weight gain. Use our BMI (Body Mass Index) table to help you. You just have to know your weight and height to calculate your weight classification.

What is Your Body Mass Index?

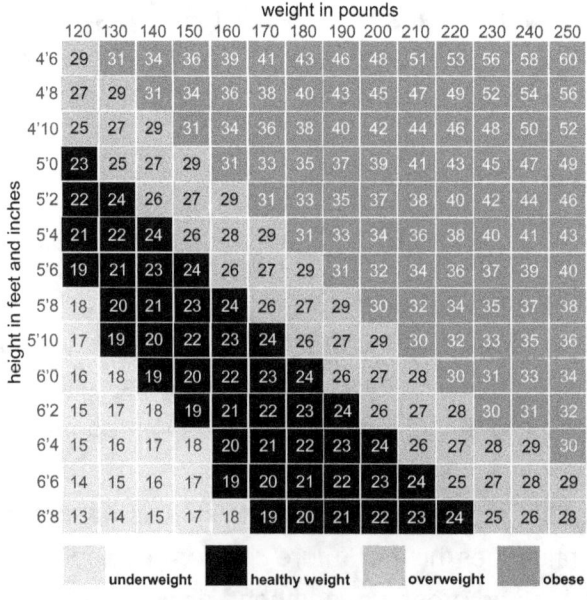

note: this chart is for adults (aged 20 years and older).

Based on your BMI weight classification, you should try to follow these recommended weight gain goals:

- **Underweight:** 28 to 40 pounds
- **Normal Weight:** 25 to 35 pounds
- **Overweight:** 11 to 20 pounds

If you gain too much weight during pregnancy, your risk of having a cesarean delivery is greater, and you may deliver a huge infant. You will also have water retention longer than other mothers after delivery.

On the other side, if you don't gain enough weight, your chances of delivering early are higher and your baby will be smaller.

> {Tip} When you are pregnant, you need to add 300 additional calories to your daily intake. You can get this by eating half a sandwich and a glass of skim milk.

What Foods to Avoid During Pregnancy

Even though you are eating for two now, you can't just consume everything you used to. There are some precautions you have to take to ensure the safety of your unborn baby. Certain foods may be perfectly fine for you but may injure the sensitive system of your little one.

It's important to learn which foods are safe to eat and which ones you should avoid. By doing this, you are providing the best possible environment for your baby to grow and develop.

Raw Meat – It is very important in pregnancy to avoid consuming raw or uncooked meat. This includes sushi and beef carpaccio. Raw or undercooked meats can contain dangerous bacteria, such as toxoplasmosis and salmonella.

Toxoplasmosis is a parasitic infection that you can get after consuming raw or undercooked meat that has been contaminated. The most common ways you become infected include working in the garden without gloves, changing the cat litter box, and eating raw or undercooked meat or fish.

If your growing baby becomes infected with toxoplasmosis, he/she may not have any symptoms at birth but can develop serious disabilities, such as blindness or mental disability later in life. In some circumstances, a new-born can display serious brain and eye damage at birth.

Deli Meats – Prepared meats, like those available at a deli counter, should be avoided when you are pregnant, unless you reheat them until they are steaming hot. These include hot dogs, smoked seafood, and luncheon meats (such as turkey, beef, and chicken). These deli meats can be con-taminated with a bacteria called listeria—which can cause miscarriage or stillborn births.

Imported Soft Cheeses – Like deli meat, imported unpasteurized cheeses can also carry listeria. Cheeses such as blue cheese, feta, Brie, or Cam-embert should be avoided. If you are a cheese fanatic, don't worry! You can still consume soft cheeses pasteurized with milk. Be sure to read package labels to find out if a product is pasteurized or not.

Undercooked Eggs – Consuming raw or undercooked eggs can be dan-gerous to your baby. Raw eggs may contain the bacteria salmonella. Like listeria, salmonella can cause miscarriage and occasionally, stillbirths. Raw eggs are often included in many commercial products, like Egg Nog and Caesar salad dressing. Remember to read package labels carefully before consuming any of these products.

If you love eggs, remember to always keep your eggs refrigerated; don't use eggs that are cracked; wash all your utensils that have had contact with raw eggs; eat eggs immediately after you cook them; foods that con-tain eggs should always be refrigerated; and don't eat foods made with raw eggs, like Hollandaise Sauce.

Signs of salmonella food poisoning include fever, abdominal cramps, and diarrhea.

Fish – Eating fish and shellfish can be important to a healthy and balanced diet, because they are good sources of high-quality protein and other nutrients. But certain kinds of fish should be avoided due to their high mercury content, which can harm your baby's nervous system. These include shark, swordfish, king mackerel, and tilefish. Canned tuna should also be avoided because of its high levels of mercury contamination.

It is generally safe to eat up to 12 ounces of other fish (two to three meals) a week, but vary the type of fish and shellfish you consume. It is safe to eat one or two servings of salmon, sardines, herring, or bluefish every month.

Caffeine – While a small amount of caffeine may provide a lift for pregnant moms, caffeine in general should be avoided. High amounts of caffeine consumption has been linked to birth defects and an increased risk of miscarriage.

Because caffeine is added to everyday food items—such as chocolate, tea, and soda—you may want to play it safe and avoid caffeine completely in the first 12 weeks of your pregnancy. Daily caffeine intake of more than 5 cups of coffee (500 mg) per day has been proven to double the risk of spontaneous miscarriage.

Alcohol – Drinking alcohol during pregnancy can be harmful to your baby's development. The degree of harm depends on how much alcohol you have consumed. Alcohol has the greatest effect during early pregnancy when many of the baby's organs are forming, but drinking at any point in the pregnancy can also cause problems.

If you had a drink or two before you realized you were pregnant, most likely, you did not harm your baby. But stop drinking now. Every time that you drink, your baby does too. Although there is no determined level of alcohol consumption that is considered safe during pregnancy, daily consumption of alcohol in early pregnancy can cause fetal alcohol syndrome – a disorder that causes growth, physical, and mental problems in the baby.

{**Fact**} Alcohol also increases the chance of a miscarriage and a pre-term baby. Alcohol abuse during pregnancy is the leading cause of mental retardation in babies.

NORMAL CHANGES TO EXPECT

Emotional Changes

Pregnancy is a time of great change. Not only is your body undergoing drastic change as your child grows inside you, but sometimes your emotional well-being can take a hit. You may be ecstatic and full of joy one second, sad and crabby the next. This whirlwind of emotions – good and bad – is absolutely normal and is due in part by fluctuation of pregnancy hormones and stress.

Share how you're feeling with your partner and loved ones, and ask for their support during this life-changing event.

As their due date approaches, many pregnant women and their partners begin to feel a bit anxious and start to worry about everything—fears about a healthy pregnancy, labor and delivery, the effect the new baby will have on their new life, and being a good parent. You can calm your fears by educating yourself on what to expect.

If you are worried about labor and delivery, take a childbirth class with your partner, so you can learn about relaxation methods and ways to manage labor pain. In addition, many hospitals offer 1 or 2 day classes on newborn care. You can also read up on how to care for your new infant during your pregnancy. All these methods, in conjunction with rest and relaxation, will help ease your mind and anxiety.

Although mood swings are a normal symptom of pregnancy for most women, pregnancy and motherhood can increase vulnerability to some mental illnesses—like depression—in some women. One in 10 pregnant women suffer depression that doesn't go away after the baby is delivered.

Being pregnant can cause certain mental illnesses to worsen or cause emotional problems to reoccur. It is possible that this is due to hormonal changes and stress. Women who have a history of depression may relapse and need special care.

Because some of the symptoms of depression (fatigue, changes in appetite, and sleeping pattern disturbances) are similar to normal pregnancy-related changes, doctors may fail to diagnose and treat depression in pregnant women.

Feeling a bit blue now and then during pregnancy is normal, but if you are sad most of the time for at least two weeks and have other symptoms of depression – including suicidal thoughts, loss of interest in work and other activities, trouble paying attention, and having aches and pains that don't get better with treatment—you should consult your doctor immediately.

Morning Sickness

Between 50 to 90 percent of pregnant women experience some degree of morning sickness – pregnancy-related nausea with or without vomiting. Remember that "morning sickness" doesn't just happen in the morning; it can occur at any point during the day. Eighty percent of pregnant women with morning sickness experience it throughout the day.

If you are experiencing nausea, gagging, vomiting, or an aversion to food, then you have morning sickness. Don't worry—mild cases of nausea and throwing up won't hurt your baby. It'll eventually end and you'll be able to eat and feel better.

The onset of morning sickness symptoms tends to be around 5 or 6 weeks with a peak at 9 weeks. It should go away in the second trimester.

Researchers are not 100 percent sure what causes morning sickness, but it is believed that the increased levels of hormones in your body during pregnancy may play a part.

To ease your nausea and vomiting, you may want to take a supplement of vitamin B6; eat dry toast or crackers in the morning before you get out of bed; get plenty of fresh air (a short walk outdoors might do you some good); drink plenty of fluids throughout the day; eat frequently (You don't want to let your stomach get empty. Be sure to eat foods that are low fat and easy to digest); and take your prenatal vitamins before bed with a snack.

COMPLICATIONS DURING PREGNANCY

Hyperemesis Gravidarum (Severe Morning Sickness)

Morning sickness should go away in the second trimester. In rare cases, less than 2 percent of pregnancies, this pregnancy-related nausea and vomiting can become so severe that you begin to lose weight and you are unable to keep down any food or fluids. This severe morning sickness is called hyperemesis gravidarum.

Hyperemesis gravidarum is the leading cause of hospitalization during early pregnancy.

Some pregnant women have a higher risk for developing this complication. These include women carrying multiples, women with a family history of hyperemesis gravidarum, those carrying a girl fetus, those who have experienced this severe morning sickness in other pregnancies, and women with a history of motion sickness or migraines.

Because women who suffer from severe morning sickness experience excessive vomiting, they are often hospitalized with dehydration. To treat them, they are given fluids through an IV line and with a round of anti-nausea medications. Most often, they do not receive any food until the vomiting stops.

The cause of severe morning sickness is not known, but several theories have been developed. These include elevated pregnancy hormones, decreased gastric motility (the food sits in your stomach and doesn't digest correctly, causing indigestion and pressure), and emotional turmoil (you have a hesitancy about your pregnancy that you are not voicing, so your feelings are converted into severe vomiting).

> **{Fun Fact}** Almost all women who suffer from severe vomiting during pregnancy completely recover and gain adequate weight for a happy outcome!

If you had to be re-admitted to the hospital on multiple occasions for severe morning sickness and you did not gain the recommended amount of weight, there's a small chance that your baby will weigh less than normal.

> **{Fact}** If you experience hyperemesis gravidarum during this pregnancy, you have a 15 to 20 percent chance of it recurring in your next pregnancy.

Urinary Tract Infections

Urinary tract infections (UTI) are one of the most common medical issues that expectant moms face. Like its name suggests, it is a bacteria infection that starts in your urinary system – which is made up of your bladder, kidneys, ureters (the tubes that connect your bladder to the kidneys), and uretha (the tube that carries the urine from your bladder to outside your body).

Between 2 to 7 percent of pregnant women have UTIs but display no classic symptoms – which include a burning sensation when you urinate. They only discover they are infected after a urine sample is tested at their doctor's office. One of the symptoms of a UTI – a strong and persistent need to urinate – is often mistaken for a common pregnancy symptom.

Urinary tract infections can lead to an increased risk of a preterm birth and low birth weight. Receiving treatment for your UTI reduces the risks of these complications.

You are normally treated for UTIs with antibiotics. These antibiotics have a proven track record to be safe for pregnant women.

WEEK 7

Prepare for an emotional rollercoaster!

Letter from Dr. James Brann · · · · · · · · · · · · · · · · ·

Week 7 brings lots of excitement! Not only are your emotions going crazy as the pregnancy hormone levels in your body increase, but you'll be having your first prenatal visit next week.

Questions may be starting to build up in your mind – Are these symptoms normal? Can my husband come with me on my first prenatal visit? Do I need to bring a videotape to record my first ultrasound? Can you prescribe me anti-nausea medicine before my visit? In my practice, my receptionist would be bombarded with questions such as these.

This rollercoaster of emotions is a normal occurrence of pregnancy, despite how unpleasant they may be for your partner and those around you.

The best part of this week – your baby is now about the size of a small blueberry. He/she is also developing more prominent facial features and will soon look like a tiny person!

Best Wishes,

James Brann m.d.

· ·

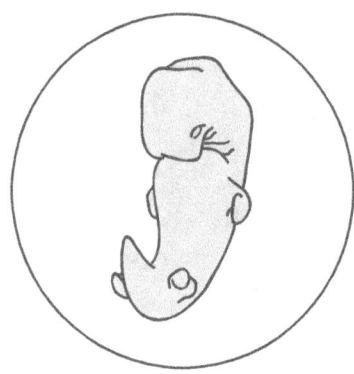

FETAL DEVELOPMENT

This week, your baby is making great strides toward looking more like a tiny person. Not only are your little one's facial features becoming more prominent, but he/she is now up to 13 mm (0.5 inches) in length from crown to rump—about the same size as a blueberry or small grape!

Your baby's brain continues to expand this week. By week 7, your little one's brain has divided into five sections—each controlling different functions, such as thought, learning, memory, speech, vision, hearing, voluntary movement, and problem solving. The head now accounts for one-third of the baby's total size.

The kidneys and lungs are starting to develop this week.

Your little blueberry's heartbeat has grown to 132 beats per minute. In its short lifetime, the baby has a running total of 2,469,600 heartbeats!

This is the week that your baby develops hand plates—a source of cells that will eventually form its tiny hands.

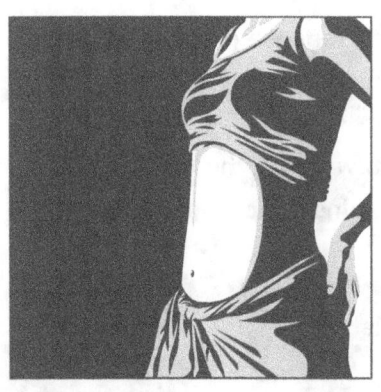

MOM'S PREGNANCY SYMPTOMS

While you still won't look very pregnant at 7 weeks, your partner may start noticing slight changes in your body. By now, your favorite jeans are probably a little uncomfortable. You may still be experiencing morning sickness. If you haven't already, you should call your doctor for an obstetrician appointment.

Food cravings begin to appear now. It is very normal for pregnant women to experience cravings as their pregnancy progresses. Food cravings may happen just because you're pregnant, but they can also occur when your body is lacking in certain nutrients. So if you're craving fruits and vegetables, eat up! Many vegetarians find that they eat meat for the first time when they are pregnant, because their bodies crave the iron that is in red meat.

Headaches are common when you are pregnant. Some women can develop migraine headaches; others just experience more headaches than normal. Pregnancy hormones, hunger, and stress all contribute to this phenomenon. Luckily, headache frequency tends to ease up after the first trimester. You may want to consult your doctor for safe treatment options. More natural methods of relieving headaches include resting in a dark, quiet room; massaging your temples; and placing a cold washcloth on your forehead.

During this week, you may experience dizziness or lightheadedness. Typically, this is a common symptom of pregnancy and should not cause too much concern.

PREGNANCY 411

Alcohol, Tobacco, and Drug Use

As a pregnant woman, you are "eating for two." Everything that you eat, drink, or consume can affect your baby's well being. That's why your lifestyle choices are so critical during pregnancy. These include trying to kick any drinking, smoking, or drug habits that you may have.

Alcohol Abuse

This was touched on in last week's chapter (week 6) under "What Foods To Avoid During Pregnancy." Although we do not know how much alcohol it takes to harm the baby growing inside you, experts agree that it is best not to drink at all during pregnancy. Not only does alcohol increase your chance of a miscarriage and delivering a preterm baby, alcohol abuse is the leading cause of mental retardation in babies.

When you drink alcohol, it quickly reaches your little one. As an adult, your liver can break down the alcohol you drink, but your baby's liver is not developed enough to do this. Therefore, alcohol is much more harmful to your little one than it is to you. The more you drink during pregnancy, the greater the danger it poses to your child.

{**Fact**} Alcohol consumption has the greatest effect during early pregnancy because many of your baby's vital organs are developing.

Heavy drinking during pregnancy can result in fetal alcohol syndrome – a disorder characterized by major physical, mental, and behavior problems. Smoking, drug use, and a poor diet can also contribute to the problems that a baby with fetal alcohol syndrome has.

Babies with fetal alcohol syndrome can have small bodies, problems with joints and limbs (known as clubfoot), heart defects, abnormal facial features, behavior problems—such as hyperactivity, anxiety, poor attention span, and low IQs. Some babies with the syndrome exhibit all these signs while others only have one or two.

{**Fact**} No types of alcohol are considered safe to drink. One beer, a shot of liquor, a mixed drink, or a glass of wine all contain approximately the same amount of alcohol and can be harmful to your baby.

If you had a drink or two before you knew you were pregnant, chances are it did not harm your baby. But you should stop drinking now.

Smoking During Pregnancy

You should not smoke or become exposed to secondhand smoke while you are pregnant. If a pregnant woman smokes, her baby is exposed to harmful chemicals like tar, nicotine, and carbon monoxide. Nicotine can cause your blood vessels to constrict, meaning your baby receives fewer nutrients and less oxygen. Carbon monoxide also lowers the amount of oxygen your baby gets.

Smoking has been linked with an increased risk for ectopic pregnancies (the baby begins to develop outside the uterus), vaginal bleeding, problems with the way the placenta attaches to the uterus, still births, and low weight babies.

Smoking and exposure to secondhand smoke can also increase your risk for:

• **Infertility** – Smoking delays conception, and increases a woman's risk of being infertile by 30 percent.

• **Placental Abruption** – A potentially serious and dangerous pregnancy complication that can occur in the third trimester, when your placenta separates from the uterine lining (the cells that line your womb). It can cause vaginal bleeding, uterine tenderness, rapid contractions, and fetal heart rate abnormalities.

• **Preterm Premature Rupture of Membranes (PPROM)** – Your water breaks before your due date or the onset of real labor.

• **Placenta Previa** – When your placenta grows in the lowest part of your womb and covers either partially or completely the opening of your uterus.

{**Fact**} Smoking can hurt the baby after birth too. Breathing in secondhand smoke can increase your newborn's risk for developing asthma and dying from sudden infant death syndrome (SIDS).

The less you smoke during pregnancy, the less harm it will do to your baby. If you cannot stop this addictive habit, cutting down on your daily cigarette intake is better than not stopping at all.

Quitting before you get pregnant is the best option for you and your baby. If you can kick the habit while you are pregnant, it is possible that you'll be able to kick it permanently. You and your family will be healthier as a result.

Abusing Illegal Drugs

Abusing illegal drugs during pregnancy is both harmful to you and your growing baby. These drugs reach the baby by crossing your placenta through your blood stream. Like with alcohol, when you take drugs, your baby is taking drugs too.

Using illegal substances during pregnancy can affect your baby in different ways, depending on what kind of drug, how much and how often you use it, and when you take it during your pregnancy. When abusing two or more illegal drugs at the same time, it is hard to predict how harmful it will be to your baby. Drugs can add and even increase each other's effects.

If you abuse illegal drugs in the early stages of pregnancy, when your baby's main body parts are developing, you increase the chances of miscarriage and birth defects. In the last trimester, drug use can stunt your baby's growth and cause premature births and stillbirths.

After the baby is born and you continue to use illegal drugs, the drugs can still be passed through your breast milk. You should stop abusing these drugs before you get pregnant.

With the widespread problem of illegal drug use in this country, there are many types of drugs out there – all are harmful to your baby during pregnancy.

• **Marijuana** - When you smoke, the active compound in marijuana can stay in your body for weeks, and exposes your baby to harmful substances in the smoke that you've inhaled. Smoking marijuana releases carbon monoxide in your body, which prevents your baby from getting enough oxygen.

• **Methamphetamine** - Commonly known as "meth," this drug raises your blood pressure and heart rate as well as putting your baby at an increased risk of miscarriage, premature birth, brain damage, and stroke. Meth can also cause placental abruption and stillbirths. Babies exposed to meth can grow too slowly in your womb. After they are born, meth-babies can have tremors, be very fussy, and have a hard time bonding with others.

• **Cocaine** - Like smoking and meth abuse, using cocaine can also cause placental abruption, so you're at higher risk for bleeding, preterm births, and delivering stillborns. Babies born to cocaine-addicted moms develop slower than other babies, and they tend to be more irritable and fussy than babies not exposed to cocaine in the womb. Other issues they may face include cocaine withdrawal, brain defects, and long term behavioral, emotional, and learning problems.

• **Ecstasy** - Similar to meth and cocaine abuse, these babies can experience mood changes, sleep problems, and loss of appetite. If you use ecstasy during pregnancy, your baby may also have long-term learning and memory problems.

• **Heroin and Narcotics** - When you use heroin during pregnancy, you have an increased risk of preterm births and delivering a stillborn. If your baby survives, they will be smaller in size and have low birth weight, have problems thinking clearly, face behavioral problems and delays in their development, and they may have a heroin or narcotic addiction.

• **"T's and Blues"** - The street name for the mix of a prescription drug and an over-the-counter allergy medication. Babies of mothers addicted to "T's and Blues" are more likely to grow more slowly in the womb and face withdrawal symptoms after birth.

• **PCP** - Known as "angel dust," this drug makes its user lose touch with reality. They may become violent and experience seizures, heart attacks and lung failure. Babies exposed to PCP in the womb tend to be smaller than normal, have poor control of their movements, and exhibit withdrawal symptoms.

• **Special K (Ketamine) -** This drug affects its user in the same way that PCP does. Babies exposed to Special K can have behavioral and learning problems.

• **LSD ("Acid") -** LSD can cause its user to hallucinate, see things that aren't there, have flashbacks, and become violent. Using LSD during pregnancy can cause birth defects.

• **Glues and Solvents -** Inhaling glues and solvents can not only damage your liver, kidneys, bone marrow, and brain, it can also cause sudden death. If you abuse these during pregnancy, you have an increased risk of miscarriage, slow growth of the baby in the womb, and preterm births. Your baby also faces birth defects similar to alcohol-affected babies.

{**Fact**} Sadly, as many as 1 in 10 babies are born to women who used illegal drugs during pregnancy.

NORMAL CHANGES TO EXPECT

Constipation, Bloating, and Gas

At some point during your pregnancy, you will become constipated. When this happens, gas can build up in your abdomen and make you feel uncomfortable and bloated. This is a normal pregnancy change that shouldn't cause you any worry. Early in your pregnancy, bloating can come with pains that are similar to the gas pains that you experience just before your regular menstrual cycle starts.

Although you won't look very pregnant at week 7, bloating causes your tummy to pooch out a little bit, making you look further along than you really are. You may experience the sensation that you ate too much or that you're too full, but it is just the result of the gas buildup in your intestines. When you are pregnant, you have more gas in your bowels because your peristalsis process – the process that moves food through your digestive system and pushes the waste out of your body – slows down. This gives you a buildup of gas, resulting in constipation and bloating.

Toward the end of your pregnancy, bloating and gas can be extremely painful as the weight of your uterus is putting pressure on your lower abdomen.

If you have constipation and gas during pregnancy, take stool softeners instead of laxatives. Natural ways for gas relief include drinking plenty of fluids (at least eight glasses of water may help); eating high fiber foods—including raw fruits, vegetables, beans, whole-grain bread, and bran cereal; and exercising regularly.

{**Fact**} **Iron supplements can worsen your constipation.**

Frequent Urination

The need to urinate more often is an almost universal pregnancy symptom that many women experience. There are several reasons for this.

First, because hydration is so important during pregnancy, expectant moms tend to drink more liquids. Second, when you are pregnant, your kidneys work super hard to flush out your body's waste products. As a result, you make more trips to the bathroom.

Third, as you progress in your pregnancy, your uterus grows larger and adds extra pressure on your bladder, making it feel like it's full when it may be nearly empty. By mid-pregnancy, some of this pressure should be relieved because your uterus is no longer pressing down on your bladder.

In the final weeks of your pregnancy, your baby "drops" into your pelvis – called "lightning." When this happens, his/her head moves down into the pelvis and presses against your cervix and bladder. This may also increase your need to go to the bathroom. Most women wake up in the middle of the night to urinate.

Having to use the bathroom frequently can be a nuisance, but unfortunately, there is not much you can do except cut back on your coffee, tea, and cola intake. These drinks contain caffeine, which make you have to urinate more often.

Do not cut back on your water intake! Drinking less to try to reduce your trips to the bathroom will rob your body of vital fluids.

{Tip} The weight of the uterus on your bladder may cause you to have urine leaks when you sneeze or cough. Wear sanitary pads or panty shields to give you extra protection.

COMPLICATIONS DURING PREGNANCY

Early Pregnancy Miscarriage

Miscarriage is the most common complication of early pregnancy. Sometimes called "spontaneous abortion," miscarriages occur in 15 to 20 percent of all pregnancies. Bleeding and strong cramping pain in the lower abdomen are common signs that a miscarriage may occur.

In a majority of cases, the cause of miscarriage is not known. When it is known, it is caused by:

• **Chromosomes** - In over 75 percent of early pregnancy miscarriages, the miscarriage is caused by a problem with the baby's chromosomes – tiny structures inside each of your cells that carry genes, which will determine your baby's physical traits. Problems with the structure of chromosomes and the number of genes they carry can result in the baby not being able to grow properly. Most of the time, these chromosomal problems are not inherited and occur by chance. Sometimes they are related to the mom's advanced age. Healthy women over age 35 have an increased risk for miscarriage.

• **Pre-existing Illnesses** - If you suffer from pre-existing illnesses – such as heart disease, uncontrolled diabetes, lupus and other autoimmune disorders, severe kidney disease linked with high blood pressure, thyroid disease, and polycystic ovary syndrome – you are at higher risk for miscarrying. Treating these illnesses before you get pregnant can decrease your risk. Some illnesses may require special care, and you may have to be closely monitored during your pregnancy.

• **Hormonal Imbalance** - Early in pregnancy, you can miscarry if you have low levels of progesterone in your body – the hormone that helps support the pregnancy to continue. Your obstetrician can administer vaginal suppositories of progesterone, but the benefits of this have not been established.

• **Uterine Problems** - Problems with the shape of your uterus (an abnormally shaped uterus such as a heart-shaped uterus instead of a regular pear-shaped one) or cervix (an incompetent cervix) can lead to miscarriage. An incompetent cervix opens without contractions or any other sign of labor.

• **Substance Use** - Smoking, heavy alcohol use, and illegal drug use during pregnancy can increase your risk of miscarriage. High levels of caffeine consumption have also been linked to an increase risk of miscarriage.

• **History of Miscarriages** - Having a miscarriage in the past can increase your risk for future miscarriages.

Warning signs that a miscarriage may occur include spotting or bleeding that can be accompanied with pain, heavy or constant bleeding with abdominal pain or cramping, and vaginal discharge without pain or bleeding.

Having a miscarriage can be very distressing, but in most cases, you did not do anything to cause your miscarriage. There has been no evidence that working, exercising, continuing to have sex, or using birth control pills before getting pregnant increases your risk.

{**Fact**} A majority of miscarriages occur within the first three months of pregnancy. Eighty percent occur within the first 12 weeks.

Repetitive Miscarriages - Antiphospholipid Syndrome

Your risk of recurrent miscarriage increases with each miscarriage you have. Sometimes multiple miscarriages can be caused by antiphospholipid syndrome – an autoimmune disorder in which your body produces high levels of the antiphospholipid antibody. An autoimmune disorder is a condition that happens when your immune system attacks and destroys healthy body tissue.

If left untreated, antiphospholipid syndrome can be life-threatening to the mother and her unborn baby as it can cause blood clots to form in the mother's arteries and veins. During pregnancy, blood clots can develop in your placenta and cause slow fetal growth, fetal distress, premature births, still births, and miscarriages.

To diagnose antiphospholipid syndrome, doctors use a combination of testing and clinical experience.

> {**Fact**} 10 to 20 percent of women with recurrent miscarriages have antiphospholipid syndrome. It is believed that 1 to 5 percent of the general population has this disorder.

Although there is no cure for this disorder, it can be treated. Pregnant women with antiphospholipid syndrome are treated with daily injections of blood thinners (Heparin) and low dose aspirin. This significantly increases the baby's survival rate. The baby's survival rate with treatment is now around 80 percent, as opposed to the 1980s when it was only 20 percent.

Vanishing Twin Syndrome

Within the first 7 weeks of pregnancy, you can miscarry and never know it. Many pregnancies can start out with two babies, but one baby will die in the womb and be reabsorbed. Without the help of an ultrasound, you would never know that your pregnancy started out with twins.

In a majority of the vanishing twin cases, you do not experience any miscarriage symptoms. If you do have vaginal bleeding, it is very light.

Often called "vanishing twin syndrome," it is very common in the early weeks of pregnancy. In a majority of the cases, your remaining twin will continue to develop without any problems.

Vanishing twins can also occur in other multiple pregnancies – triples, quadruplets, quintuplets, and so on.

Vanishing twin syndrome is often diagnosed at the doctor's office. You may undergo a routine ultrasound early in your pregnancy, and two babies are detected. Later, when you return to the doctor, only one twin can be detected on the ultrasound. The other twin has "vanished."

The causes of this phenomenon are not known. It may be caused by chromosomal defects in the vanishing twin.

Your first prenatal
visit is this week!

Letter from Dr. James Brann • • • • • • • • • • • • • • • • • •

What an exciting week you have ahead of you! Not only is this the week that you may have your first prenatal visit, but soon, you will get to see your little one's heartbeat on an ultrasound.

Once the doctor officially confirms your pregnancy, he/she will talk to you about starting on prenatal vitamins and changing your eating habits to ensure your baby gets all the proper nutrients he/she needs. If you have special diet restrictions, including a vegan or vegetarian diet, be sure to mention this to your doctor so he/she can help supplement your meals. In this chapter, under "Pregnancy 411," I offer some invaluable tips and advice on how to resolve vitamin and nutrient deficiencies in vegetarian diets with some minor dietary changes.

If this is your first prenatal visit, you may still be experiencing light spotting or bleeding. This may be due to many reasons, including implantation bleeding, threatened miscarriage, an infection, cervical polyps, and more. If the bleeding worries you, contact your physician immediately. We will discuss the many reasons for spotting or bleeding in early pregnancy in this week.

Don't be surprised if you soon start to develop food cravings, food aversions, indigestion, or heartburn. These are all normal pregnancy symptoms

and should not cause you any concern.

**Your baby is undergoing some delightful changes this week – including his/
her hands becoming more distinct, nipples starting to form, and bones beginning to develop.**

Best Wishes,

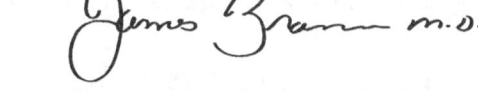

FETAL DEVELOPMENT

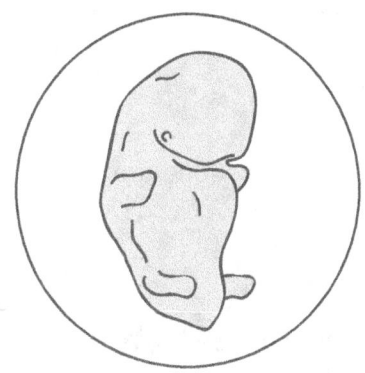

By week 8 of your pregnancy, your little one
has grown to 0.63 inches – about the size of
a lima bean. With every week that passes,
he or she is hurling toward becoming a rec-
ognizable human being.

Your baby's heartbeat is up to 151 beats per
minute. By the end of this week, his or her
heart will have beaten 1,522,080 times!

By now, the cerebral hemispheres of the baby's brain are growing consid-
erably faster than other sections. Nerve cells are starting to connect with
each other.

{**Fun Fact**} Did you know that the tip of your baby's nose has
formed by week 8?

By the middle of this week, your little one's elbows are distinct.

"Ossification" or bone formation begins this week. Your baby's collarbone
and the bones of the upper and lower jaw are developing.

By now, your baby will start making spontaneous, reflexive movements to promote his/her normal neuromuscular development – the muscles and nerves that work together to regulate movement.

Blood cell formation is underway at this stage in pregnancy. Your little one's liver is forming lymphocytes – a type of white blood cell that is key in developing a healthy immune system.

During this time, the external ear of your child is beginning to take shape.

By week 8, the diaphragm, the primary muscle that you use when you breathe, is already formed.

Your baby's hand plates, which began developing a couple of weeks ago, are starting to flatten and look more like a hand.

Nipples have begun to appear along the side of the chest and are working their way to their final location.

MOM'S PREGNANCY SYMPTOMS

Although you still won't look very pregnant at week 8, you may appear "chubby" to people who don't know you are pregnant. Your uterus, which started as the size of a small lemon pre-pregnancy, has expanded to the size of a large orange or small grapefruit!

By now, you're probably battling morning sickness symptoms and fatigue – which is heightened in your first trimester. You may also notice some mild abdominal cramping, which is a very common experience and will continue for several weeks.

Lower backaches, which are another common pregnancy symptom, may start to plague you this week. Backaches are the result of your uterus applying pressure to the lower part of your spine. If you experience a sharp pain in your buttocks and along the side of your thigh, don't be alarmed. This is just your uterus placing pressure on the sciatic nerve that attaches to your buttocks and the side of your leg.

By now, you may be anxious to share the news of your miracle with those around you. This is a personal choice. Some women can't wait to tell everyone the news, while others prefer to wait later in the pregnancy when there is less chance for miscarriage or when they start showing.

PREGNANCY 411

Diet Restrictions During Pregnancy

As we covered in Week 5, proper nutrition and a balanced diet are incredibly important to the health of you and your unborn baby. Because the foods you eat are the main source of nutrition for your baby, you have to be conscious about maintaining a balanced and healthy diet.

During pregnancy, please do not diet as a way to keep the pregnancy pounds off. When you do this, essential nutrients end up being left out of your meals and this can hurt your baby's development.

You may want to limit your consumption of certain types of fish, caffeine intake, unwashed fruits and vegetables, unpasteurized dairy products, and undercooked meats. Foods to avoid in pregnancy were explored in Week 6.

Junk Food

If you have cravings for junk food, it's okay to give into these occasionally. Just be careful that it doesn't overtake your diet. Junk food may comfort and fill you up fast, but they are empty calories – high in fat and low in the vitamins and nutrients that your baby needs. Most junk food is low in vitamins A and C, folic acid, fiber, and calcium – all of which are very important in preventing birth defects and ensuring that your baby develops properly.

> {Tip} Snacking and eating small healthy meals throughout the day is a good way to get the extra calories and nutrients you need, and it will help your morning sickness and heartburn.

Eating Out

When you eat out, try to look for whole grain foods, fruits, vegetables, and calcium-rich foods. Other tips for a healthier diet while eating out include:

• If you order sandwiches, opt for grilled or charbroiled meats rather than the breaded and deep-fried alternatives. Limit your intake of cheese, bacon, and mayonnaise.

• For side dishes, choose a baked potato instead of French fries, and steamed vegetables if available.

• If you are a pizza lover, order thin-crust pizzas baked with low-fat cheeses and vegetables or low-fat meats. Avoid high-fat meats like sausage and pepperoni.

• Order salads that are free of fat-containing dressings, bacon bits, and shredded cheese.

• Add fresh fruits, vegetables, and beans to give you more fiber, vitamins, and minerals.

• If you are craving dessert, go for low-fat frozen yogurt cones or sundaes and fresh fruit rather than fried pies and cookies.

Vegetarian and Vegan Diets

If you are a vegetarian or vegan, you can continue your diet throughout your pregnancy but you will need to plan your meals carefully so that you get all the nutrients that your baby needs to grow.

Vegetarian diets, especially vegan ones that exclude all animal products, may not contain sufficient amounts of essential amino acids, iron, trace minerals, vitamin B-12, vitamin D, calcium, or complex lipids to maintain a healthy pregnancy. Also, because vegetarian diets lack the proper nutrients, meeting the energy requirements that your body needs during pregnancy can be difficult.

These vitamin and nutrient deficiencies can be resolved with minor dietary changes, such as:

• Supplement your diet with other non-meat and non-diary protein sources, such as nuts, peanut butter, legumes, soy products, and tofu.

• To get enough Vitamin D in your body, you can consume fortified milk, eggs, and fish. If you are a vegan, you can either take a supplement or spend 10 to 15 minutes in direct sunlight three times a week.

• Eat or drink at least four servings of calcium-rich foods a day to ensure that you get 1200 mg of calcium. These foods include dairy products, seafood, leafy green vegetables, tofu, and dried beans or peas.

• You need to get 27 mg of iron in your daily diet, so be sure to consume enriched grain products (like rice), eggs, leafy green vegetables, broccoli, Brussels sprouts, sweet potatoes, peanuts, dried beans and peas, raisins, and prunes.

• Consume at least one source of Vitamin C every day. These include oranges, grapefruits, strawberries, honeydew, cauliflower, broccoli, green peppers, tomatoes, mustard greens, and Brussels sprouts.

• Folic acid is incredibly important during pregnancy to protect against neural tube defects. Be sure to include this in your diet. Vegetarian sources of folic acid include chickpeas, black beans, black-eyed peas, lima beans, and dark green leafy vegetables.

• Don't forget adding Vitamin A into your diet. Consume at least one source every other day. Too much vitamin A is not a good thing. These foods include carrots, pumpkins, sweet potatoes, squash, spinach, turnip greens, beat greens, apricots, and cantaloupe.

• Eat at least one source of Vitamin B12 every day. Vitamin B12 can be found in fish and shellfish, eggs, and diary products. Vegans may need to take a vitamin B12 supplement.

Lactose-Intolerance

Milk and dairy products are the best ways of getting calcium in your diet. However, some women are lactose-intolerant and cannot handle dairy products well. They may experience bloating, gas, diarrhea, and indigestion after drinking milk and consuming dairy products. These symptoms tend to improve during pregnancy.

If you are still having problems, talk to your doctor. You may be prescribed calcium supplements if you cannot get enough calcium from other food sources, such as cheese, yogurt, sardines, certain kinds of salmon, spinach and other dark green leafy vegetables, calcium-fortified soy milk and orange juice.

> {**Fact**} If you do not have sufficient amounts of calcium for your growing baby, he/she will rob it from your bones and you can end up with osteoporosis (fragile bones).

Advanced Maternal Age

Many women are deciding to have babies later and later in life. While there is no set age when it's unsafe for a woman to become pregnant, the demands that pregnancy places on the body can increase an older woman's risk for pregnancy complications. Older moms may need to visit the doctor more often, endure special tests, and need special care during their labor and delivery.

Once you reach your early 30s, fertility tends to decline. It may be harder for you to get pregnant. Often, this is due to problems with ovulation – the release of the eggs from your ovaries. As you age, ovulation occurs less frequently and your eggs are not as easily fertilized as a younger woman's. In addition, older women can experience blocked fallopian tubes and endometriosis – a disorder in which the tissue that lines your uterus grows outside your womb on your fallopian tubes or ovaries. Both these complications can cause infertility.

The father's age may also play a role in infertility. As he ages, his fertility also decreases.

{Tip} If you are over 35 and have been trying to get pregnant for more than six to ten months without any success, you may want to talk to a doctor about assisted roproductive technologies.

A woman's risk for miscarriage increases the older she gets. In many cases, these miscarriages are related to chromosomal issues.

Women over 35 also have a four to eight-fold higher chance of an ectopic pregnancy than younger women. This may be due to a number of risk factors that have accumulated over time, including previous infections or endometriosis that caused damage to the fallopian tubes and multiple sexual partners.

Your risk of delivering a baby with birth defects also increases with age. Your child may end up with a chromosome-related disease, such as Down syndrome and Spina Bifida.

In many cases, older women are offered testing for genetic disorders and other medical problems before and during pregnancy.

Older moms also have an increased risk of developing high blood pressure during pregnancy, and this can cause problems with the placenta and the growth of the baby. High blood pressure can even worsen during pregnancy.

You are also more likely to develop gestational diabetes – diabetes that occurs during pregnancy. This can lead to stillbirths and macrosomia (an overly large baby).

Despite all these risk factors, many moms who are over 35 go on to have normal, healthy children.

{**Fact**} **Studies show that pregnant women over 35 are more likely to deliver via c-sections than their younger counterparts. Older women tend to face more labor complications.**

NORMAL CHANGES TO EXPECT

Food Cravings & Aversions

We've all heard the tales of husbands driving around in the middle of the night to try to satisfy his wife's craving for pickles and ice cream. Although we laugh at these, it is very common for women to get food cravings.

No one quite knows what causes these pregnancy cravings. It may be due to your pregnancy hormones or your body's need to get extra calories into your system as it works in overdrive to support the baby growing inside you. Food cravings may also signal nutritional deficiencies. If you begin to crave chocolate, this may be a sign that you need more Vitamin B in your system. Red meat and steak cravings may signal you need more iron and protein. Substantial cravings for ice may also suggest an iron deficiency.

Instead of resisting your food cravings, it is okay to give into them some-times. Be careful not to overindulge in one type of food and neglect the rest of your diet.

Sometimes, you may get some rather bizarre cravings for non-food items such as clay, chalk, laundry starch, coffee grounds, plaster, toothpaste, and paint chips. This condition is called "pica," and it may be harmful to your pregnancy as it prevents you from getting the nutrients that you need.

Pica is caused by iron deficiency anemia – which will increase your fatigue and possibly decrease your baby's oxygen supply. Once you treat your anemia, your pica will go away.

Along with your food cravings, your pregnancy hormones can make you totally adverse to certain foods. For example, the thought of drinking milk or eating spaghetti can make you feel sick to your stomach. The smell of pizza can offend you and you can't even stand looking at one.

Most food aversions occur in the first trimester and they are accompanied by morning sickness. Most often they go away as your pregnancy progresses.

Heartburn & Indigestion

During your pregnancy, it is not uncommon for you to experience bouts of heartburn and indigestion. Be careful not to confuse the two sensations as the same thing. Heartburn is a burning sensation in your throat and chest, while indigestion makes you feel full, bloated, and gassy. Indigestion is caused by a slow-moving stomach that is taking a long time to empty.

{Fact} 30 to 50 percent of all pregnant women experience heartburn. If you had issues with heartburn before your pregnancy, you will most likely experience it while pregnant.

In the beginning of your pregnancy, heartburn and indigestion are caused by rising levels of pregnancy hormones in your body. These hormones relax the muscle valve between your throat and your stomach. Because the valve is relaxed, it doesn't close all the way and stomach acids can leak into your esophagus, giving you a burning sensation.

As your pregnancy progresses and your uterus gets larger, the uterus pushes against your stomach and intestines, slowing things down and causing you some discomfort.

Although heartburn and indigestion are annoying, they are absolutely normal and do not require medical help. They can be relieved by a few simple tricks:

• Instead of three big meals, try eating six mini-meals throughout the day. When you eat, be sure to eat at a slower pace and to chew your food well. This will help avoid that heavy sensation of eating too much too fast.

• Don't drink too much while you eat. Instead, drink between meals. Drinking too much with your meals can dilute the stomach acid that aids in digestion.

• Stay away from foods that are fried, greasy, and full of fat, as these are harder to digest.

• Avoid fizzy drinks, citrus juices/drinks, and spicy foods. These can irritate your esophagus, giving you more heartburn.

• Avoid eating or drinking before you go to bed. Try to avoid lying down right after you eat. When you lie down, the acid in your stomach can flow back up into your esophagus and give you heartburn.

• Raise the head of your bed. Ask your partner to prop a couple of books or wood blocks underneath the legs of the head of your bed. You can also stack extra pillows under your shoulders.

• Talk to your physician about using antacids and other medications to help.

COMPLICATIONS DURING PREGNANCY

Human Immunodeficiency Virus Infection (HIV)

It is estimated that about 2 out of every 1,000 pregnant women are infected with HIV (human immunodeficiency virus). This virus is spread through contact with an infected person's body fluids, such as blood and semen. Infected mothers can pass the virus to their baby through the placenta, vaginal fluids, and breast milk.

Once the virus is inside your body, HIV destroys the healthy cells that are part of your immune system, leaving you vulnerable to other diseases and infections that can ultimately kill you. When a person with HIV contracts one of these infections or has a low level of healthy immune system cells, he or she has AIDS (acquired immunodeficiency syndrome). Not everyone who is HIV positive has AIDS, though.

In many cases, a person with HIV does not immediately get sick. It may take five years or more before symptoms appear. These can include flu-like symptoms, unexplained weight loss, fatigue, swollen lymph nodes, cold sweats, fever, diarrhea, and cough.

To reduce your risk of an HIV infection, do not inject drugs; avoid having more than one sexual partner; avoid having sex with a partner who may use drugs or have other sexual partners; and be sure to use latex condoms during sex.

Although this is a life-long illness that has no cure, there are steps that you can take to stay healthy and to protect your baby from becoming infected.

Treating a mother with HIV greatly reduces the infection rate of the baby. If a pregnant women with HIV starts treatment between weeks 14 to 34 of her pregnancy, her baby has less than an 8 percent chance of getting infected, or 1 in 12. If she does not get treated, about 25 percent of the babies (1 in 4) will get the virus.

Your risk of passing the virus to your baby depends on your viral load – or how much of the virus you have in your blood.

For best outcomes, if you are HIV positive, you should continue to take your medication during pregnancy, labor, and delivery.

Like with other diseases, medications that are used to treat HIV can affect your baby's health. Stopping treatment will increase your baby's risk of infection.

Many babies who end up with HIV are usually infected around the time of delivery. During the labor and delivery process, the baby can be exposed to the mother's body fluids, i.e. the amniotic sac, which can spread the virus. If an infected woman's water breaks, her baby is at higher risk of infection. Because of this, many pregnant women with HIV are offered cesarean sections before their due date.

> **{Fact}** If you take medications for HIV during pregnancy and you undergo a scheduled cesarean delivery, your baby's risk of contracting HIV during pregnancy is only 2 percent.

Although having a c-section may be more beneficial to the baby, mothers with weaker immune systems have a higher chance of getting infections. Drugs to prevent infection may be given to these women when they deliver.

After your baby is born, he or she will be tested for HIV. Even if a baby tests positive at birth, this does not necessarily mean that your baby is HIV positive. Many babies that are not infected but test positive may still have the mother's antibodies in his or her blood. By 6 months, these antibodies disappear.

To decrease your baby's chance of becoming infected, babies of HIV-positive moms are treated with medication within 12 hours after delivery.

If you are HIV positive, you should not breast feed your child. Breast milk can pass on the virus. Infant formula is the safest way to provide your baby with the nutrients he or she needs. Because you are not breastfeeding, your breasts may become full of milk (engorged) and may hurt for several days after delivery. To relieve the pain, support your breasts in a tight bra or bind them with an elastic bandage. Apply ice and take over-the-counter pain relievers, like acetaminophen or ibuprofen. Do not apply heat to or massage your breasts, as this will increase milk production.

> **{Tip}** After your baby is born, he/she will need special care to avoid infection. Remember to not let your body fluids come into contact with your child's mouth, eyes, nose, or rectum.

Early Maternal Hemorrhage

Vaginal bleeding early on in your pregnancy can alarm you. You may have just discovered you were pregnant and you've been overwhelmed with excitement and joy. Now you are bleeding. What does this mean? Have I lost my baby?

Bleeding early in pregnancy can be serious, but other times, it is not. Please contact your physician if you have bleeding of any kind.

{**Fact**} Up to 40 percent of all pregnant women experience bleeding in the first trimester.

Early pregnancy bleeding can be caused by a number of factors, including implantation bleeding, threatened miscarriage, vanishing twin, vaginal infections, genital warts, swollen labia, cervical polyps, uterine fibroid, and sexual intercourse.

• **Implantation -** Around the time that you may be expecting your period, you may experience some implantation bleeding – blood that results from the fertilized egg attaching to the lining of your uterus. Because of the timing, you may confuse this with your menstrual blood, which is heavier in blood flow. When in doubt, a trip to your doctor's office will confirm you are pregnant.

• **Threatened Miscarriage -** Bleeding is a common sign that a miscarriage may occur. Your physician will diagnose you with a threatened miscarriage if you have vaginal bleeding accompanied with mild cramping, but an ultrasound exam shows that the baby is still moving and has a heartbeat.

{**Fact**} Threatened miscarriages are typically seen at 7 to 11 weeks. Over 90 percent of the time, the pregnancy continues without any other problems.

If you have a threatened miscarriage, you may have a few spots of bright red blood, followed by brown, coffee-ground looking material. Your doctor may recommend you avoid having sex and get extra rest, but be warned, these measures have not been proven to prevent miscarriage.

If you experience heavy bleeding and think you have passed fetal tissue, place it in a clean container and take it to your physician. He or she will do a pelvic exam to see if your cervix has opened and if a miscarriage has occurred.

• **Vanishing Twin** - We discussed this in Week 7. The term "vanishing twin" is used to describe a pregnancy that started out with two babies, but one of the babies has died early in your pregnancy. You may experience some spotting (light bleeding) and cramping with this phenomenon. In most cases, the remaining baby is fine and the pregnancy will continue as normal.

• **Vaginal Infections** - Vaginal infections are very common during pregnancy. These infections can make your vaginal tissue swollen and inflamed, causing it to be very delicate and bleed easily after a wipe or sexual intercourse. All vaginal infections, including your common yeast infection, need to be treated. Once the infection is treated, the bleeding should disappear.

• **Genital Warts** - Genital warts tend to increase in size and number during pregnancy. Pre-pregnancy, you may have noticed a few small bumps on the outside of the vagina. During your pregnancy, these will grow quite large and bleed easily. You may be concerned about the bleeding if you don't recognize that it is coming from the warts. Warts can be treated during pregnancy, and the irritation and bleeding associated with them will be minimized.

• **Swollen Labia** - Your vagina and the labia swell during pregnancy. Even the smallest amount of trauma to this area can cause it to bleed. Most often, this type of bleeding occurs from blunt trauma, such as riding a bike, or during normal sexual intercourse. Scratching can also cause your labia to bleed. Blood from your swollen labia will not harm your baby.

• **Cervical Polyp** - A cervical polyp can cause bleeding during your pregnancy. These polyps are fingerlike growths within or near the surface of your cervix. During pregnancy, these polyps can enlarge and cause bleeding during sex. Although cervical polyps will not harm your baby, your physician may take a tissue sample from it to ensure that it is not cancerous.

• **Uterine Fibroid** - Uterine fibroids, which are non-cancerous tumors that grow on the wall of your uterus, can cause bleeding during pregnancy. If you experience mild bleeding but no cramping from the fibroids, you will need to be observed by a doctor but no additional treatment is required. In this case, the risk to your baby is very minimal. The blood you may see is light and brownish in color, like old coffee grounds. If your fibroids are large, or if your baby is implanted close to the tumor, you may have a slightly increased chance of miscarriage.

• **Sexual Intercourse** - Some pregnant women complain that they experience vaginal bleeding after sex, and they are worried that the blood is coming from the baby. Don't be alarmed if you experience this – the blood is actually coming from your cervix (the opening to the womb).

During pregnancy, the surface of the cervix tends to bleed easily when touched. You can experience light bleeding after sex, but this vaginal bleeding will not harm your baby. You may continue to have sex safely unless the bleeding bothers you.

PRENATAL CARE

What to Expect at your First Prenatal Visit

Congrats! This should be the week that you will be having your first prenatal visit! Remember that this doctor's visit will be longer and more involved than future visits. It is a great time to ask any questions that you may have, discuss your concerns, and learn more about what to expect about your physician's prenatal care routine.

At this visit, be prepared to fill out a lengthy health history. Some physicians will mail you the forms ahead of time, as it may take awhile to complete. A typical health history questionnaire asks questions about:

- Your previous deliveries and complications
- Both your partner and your genetic history
- Significant previous medical problems
- Previous surgeries
- Current medications that you are on
- Allergies

- Alcohol, tobacco, and illicit drug use
- Your eating habits
- Environmental or occupational hazard exposure
- Sexually transmitted disease history
- Other gynecology history

The more information you can provide about your medical history, the better prepared your doctor will be in structuring your prenatal care and providing any special help you may need.

At your first doctor's visit, you will also have a physical exam, which includes a pap smear and pelvic exam, lab work and most likely, an ultrasound to confirm your due date. The lab tests will not only determine your blood type and Rh factor, but it screens for antibodies that could harm your baby, examines your immunity to the rubella virus (or German measles), and checks for anemia, bladder infections, sexually transmitted diseases, hepatitis B, and HIV.

The most exciting part of your first prenatal visit is that you will be able to find out your estimated date of delivery, or your due date. To calculate your due date, your doctor uses a combination of methods, including the date of your last period, an ultrasound measurement of your baby, and the date of conception, if available.

Calculating the correct due date is very important. Not only is it used as a timeline for checking the growth of your baby, your due date helps to time prenatal tests and to make sure your labor and delivery does not happen too early or too late. Most women go into labor between 37 and 42 weeks.

{**Fun Fact**} Only about 1 in 20 women actually deliver their baby on the exact due date they are given.

WEEK

9

Your first trimester will be
over before you know it!

Letter from Dr. James Brann ·

Your first trimester is chugging along and will be over before you know it. As your fatigue and morning sickness continue in full swing, just remember that relief is in sight. In a few short weeks, you will get some much needed relief from your pregnancy symptoms.

Lab results from your first prenatal visit come back this week. Some of you may be receiving a phone call from your doctor's office with the news that you had some blood work abnormalities or an abnormal pap smear. This can be a scary experience, but luckily, many of these abnormalities can be easily treated.

For a few of you, week 9 is when the initial shock of an unplanned pregnancy has sunk in and it's time for you to make a decision on whether or not you wish to continue your pregnancy. In my practice, this is the week that I receive phone calls from expectant mothers asking for my advice.

For other patients, they call me with worries concerning their due date. Perhaps they were unaware of their pregnancy and were still on the birth control pill. What does this mean for the health of their baby? This topic will also be covered under the "Complications During Pregnancy" section of this chapter.

Your little one is starting to develop his or her sex organs this week. The most amazing news – your baby's heart is almost completely developed!

Best Wishes,

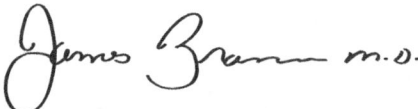

FETAL DEVELOPMENT

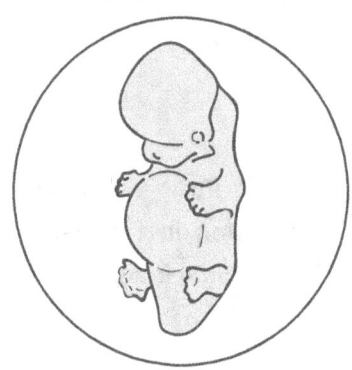

Your little one is growing up fast. His/her face is becoming more and more distinct with each day that passes! By now, all your baby's organs should be functioning on their own.

Your little one has grown to a whopping 0.90 inch – about the size of a large grape. He/she now weighs 0.07 ounce. This may not seem like a huge milestone, but just wait. Your baby will start packing on the pounds pretty soon.

By now, your little one's heart rate has reached 170 beats per minute. It should start slowly descending from here on out.

Your baby's heart is nearly complete. By 9 weeks, it should have divided into four separate chambers.

> **{Fun Fact}** Electrical activity of the heart recorded at 9 weeks reveals a similar pattern to that of an adult's!

At this point, your baby's arms, legs, head, and torso should all be in place. Your little one is looking more and more like a tiny person.

Fingers are now separate and toes are connected at the base. Your baby's hands can now come together, as can the feet!

Knee joints are also present and leg movements can be seen with ultra-sound.

The little one's eyelids are undergoing rapid growth. This week, they will fuse shut and won't open again until around 27 weeks.

The sex organs are developing now, though your healthcare provider can't tell the sex of the baby just yet. You will have to wait until 18 to 20 weeks of gestation to find out.

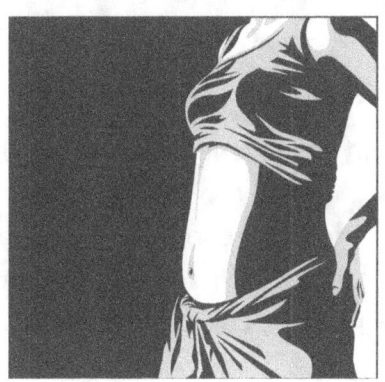

MOM'S PREGNANCY SYMPTOMS

You're probably feeling very bloated this week. The pregnancy hormones that are charging through your body may slow down your digestion, giving you bouts of constipation. As a result, gas can build up in your abdomen and cause bloating and pain. (You can read more about consitpation, bloating, and gas in Week 7's chapter under "Changes to Expect.")

By week 9, your uterus has expanded to the size of a small melon, though most women barely look pregnant. As a result of your expanding uterus, you may begin to experience a dull ache in your buttocks that won't go away. This is due to the weight of your uterus pressing against your lower spine and sciatic nerve – the nerve that travels from your lower back through your buttocks and into your leg.

You may also experience some pregnancy-related mood swings and anxiety around this time, due to rising hormones. Headaches are also common in the first trimester. For some women, these can be a minor annoyance, but for others, they can turn into extremely painful migraines.

If you've been battling morning sickness, it may be getting worse and soon become intolerable. But relief is in sight. Your second trimester is just around the corner, and for most women, this means relief from their nausea and vomiting.

The second trimester is often called the "honeymoon" stage of pregnancy. Many of your more bothersome pregnancy symptoms will be temporarily relieved until the third trimester rolls around.

{**Fun Fact**} **One misconception that many women have is that the size of your tummy equals the size of your uterus. Not so!**

PREGNANCY 411

Conception While Using the Birth Control Pill

The birth control pill is a safe and effective way to prevent pregnancy, and it is used by millions of women annually. The hormones in the pill prevent ovulation, and it thickens your cervical mucus to block sperm from entering the cervix, and thins your uterus lining so that a fertilized egg cannot attach to it. The combination of these events makes it unlikely that you will become pregnant on the pill.

If you are on the pill, you have less than a 1 in 100 chance of getting pregnant. If you end up pregnant, it may be due to a missed pill or the pill not being absorbed in your system, due to vomiting or interactions with other medications you may be on.

Although almost 99 percent effective, the pill only works if you take it correctly. Failing to take your birth control pill on a regular basis can lead to unexpected pregnancy. In the case of a missed pill, you should have a backup method of birth control, such as condoms and spermicides.

Some studies have suggested that being overweight can increase your risk of getting pregnant while on the pill, while other studies have found a weak correlation. Because of this, researchers cannot come to a consensus on whether your body weight affects the pill's effectiveness.

If you end up getting pregnant on the pill, but are unaware of the pregnancy for a while, don't worry. Inadvertent pill taking during early pregnancy has not been linked to any birth defects.

> {**Fact**} If you end up accidently conceiving due to a missed pill, emergency contraception can be used to prevent pregnancy. This includes the "morning-after pill (Plan B)."

Your Early Choices in an Unplanned Pregnancy

Although pregnancy is a blessed and exciting event for many families, unplanned pregnancies can often come as a shock. Your emotions can range from joy to ambivalence or distress. This pregnancy may come at an inconvenient time – you may feel that you are not ready to raise a child. On the other side of the spectrum, you might be delightfully surprised because you have been looking forward to motherhood for years!

If you are ready for parenthood, we hope this book will help guide you through the first trimester of your pregnancy. However, if you are facing the reality of an unexpected pregnancy, you will want information to help you make an informed decision on what to do next.

What is right for you? Keeping the baby, adoption, or termination of your pregnancy (abortion)?

Your decision will be influenced by several factors, including your health, personal values, beliefs, and current life situation.

If you haven't already been to the doctor, you should schedule an appointment right away. You want to confirm your pregnancy and see how many weeks along you are.

At your doctor's visit, come with a list of questions that you may have. These can include:

• Do I have any medical problems that pose a risk to the baby's health?

• Do you, the doctor, notice any signs that something could be wrong with the pregnancy?

• What are the limitations of my options based on how far along my pregnancy is?

• What does this choice mean for me later in life? Future pregnancies? Physical and emotional state?

> {**Tip**} **Do not make this decision alone. Seek help and advice from your husband or partner, circle of family and friends, doctors, family planning clinics, and professional counselors.**

As you are making your decision regarding your unplanned pregnancy, ask yourself these questions:

• How are you going to care for your newborn? Do you have a partner and family members that are willing to share the responsibility of raising a baby?

• Babies are a 24-hour responsibility, and they require a lot of work. Do you have the emotional and physical stamina to manage your new role as a parent?

• Can you financially handle the cost of raising a child? (Data shows that the average American will spend a couple hundred thousand dollars on raising a child from infancy to adulthood.)

• Parenthood can be a very rewarding experience, but it will also affect your relationship, social life, and career. Are you willing to accept how being a parent will change your lifestyle?

If you end up deciding to continue your pregnancy and raise your child, you will want to start prenatal care as soon as possible. The earlier you start prenatal care, the healthier your baby will be and the smoother your pregnancy will progress.

If you want to deliver your baby, but you do not want to raise him/her, adoption is a great option! You may worry about your ability to provide and care for your child, and you want to give your little one a better life.

Because adoption is a permanent decision, it should not be taken lightly or considered too quickly. Give yourself plenty of time to think and make your decision. Talk to your partner, family, and friends about the possibility of placing your child up for adoption. Ask for their thoughts and feelings, but remember that the ultimate decision is yours.

Before making the decision to adopt, ask yourself these questions:

- Can you be a mother or are you just "not ready?"

- Can you manage the emotions and feelings that come with giving up your baby?

- What about your partner? Is he supportive in this decision?

If you decide to go through the adoption process, be prepared for the legal work and emotions It brings. The first thing you need to do to start the adoption process is to contact an adoption agency or an adoption lawyer.

Next, the lawyer or adoption agency will help you create an adoption plan. This plan allows you to influence the various stages of the adoption process. You can choose the adoptive parents; determine if you want contact with them; if you want them present at the baby's birth; and if you want to see your baby after he/she is born.

After the adoption plan is complete, the next step is to let the lawyer know when you are going to the hospital to deliver. After your baby is born, you and the baby's birth father will sign the final papers, and the baby will go home with his/her new parents.

There are three types of adoptions that you can choose from:

• **Open Adoption:** You meet the potential adoptive family prior to the birth. You have access to the adoptive family's contact information. You and your adoptive family can choose to meet and remain in contact throughout your child's lifetime. You may be able to see your child grow up, not as a parent but in an "extended family" type of relationship. In open adoptions, your child will grow up knowing they are loved by their family members – both their birth parents and their adoptive ones.

• **Semi-Open Adoption:** You choose the adoptive family through written profiles. You will only know the adoptive parents' first names. A third party will mediate contact between you and the adoptive parents before and after your baby's birth. After birth, meetings are arranged through a mediator. You do not have direct contact with your child throughout his/her lifetime, but the adoptive parents will sometimes update you on your child's life via letters and pictures.

• **Closed/Confidential Adoption:** You allow the adoption agency to choose your baby's adoptive family. You do not have contact with the adoptive family or with your child at all.

{**Fact**} According to the National Survey of Family Growth, less than one percent of children born to single moms were placed for adoption between 1989 and 1995.

If you decide you do not want to continue with your pregnancy, your physician may perform an abortion ("induced abortion"). An abortion is usually performed before week 12 of your pregnancy.

Induced abortions are either done by surgery or with medication. Your doctor should explain all the risks that come with each type.

The longer you wait to make your decision to have an induced abortion, the more complications and risks you face.

As with all surgeries, abortions come with some physical risks. These include hemorrhaging (bleeding), infection, damage to the uterus, and maternal death. Maternal death from abortion is low, but it is lowest before 8 weeks. The risk factor increases after 18 weeks.

Women who undergo abortions may experience a range of emotions afterwards, including relief, guilt, sadness, and a sense of loss. Though no evidence from large surveys link abortions to an increased risk of subsequent depression, abortions are a serious matter and should not be taken lightly.

{**Fact**} Close to 50 percent of pregnancies in the U.S. are unexpected, and almost one-half of these end up in abortions.

NORMAL CHANGES TO EXPECT

Headaches

Headaches are very common during pregnancy. Pregnancy hormones, hunger, and stress can all contribute to this symptom. Over 90 percent of pregnancy headaches are migraine and tension headaches.

Most women with a history of migraine headaches report that their headaches improved during pregnancy. Less than 5 percent claim their migraines worsened. If you have never had a migraine headache before, it can develop for the first time in your first trimester. Recurrent migraine headaches typically rear their ugly heads around the third trimester.

{**Fact**} Migraines affect 18 percent of all American women. Only 6 or 7 percent of sufferers are men.

Pregnant women have to be careful about what medications they take to treat their migraine and tension headaches. Certain drugs that are effective in non-pregnant women can have harmful effects on your growing baby.

Many doctors suggest taking acetaminophen (Tylenol) for your migraines. Acetaminophen will not hurt your pregnancy or your baby.

Whether treated or untreated, pregnant women with headaches go on to have healthy babies.

{Tip} For headache relief without medication, you may want to place a cold washcloth on your forehead, gently massage your temples, or rest in a dark, quiet room.

Fatigue

In your first trimester, expect to feel worn-out and tired. As your body's production of progesterone soars, your body is spending all of its energy creating and supporting your growing baby. Your body is also increasing its blood production to carry nutrients to your little one, and this can really sap up your energy. If you've been struggling with bouts of morning sickness, this can also contribute to your exhaustion.

Luckily, relief is in sight. Most women report that their fatigue gets better during the second trimester. However, energy levels will drop again in the third trimester, because of all that additional weight that you are carrying around. In the latter part of your pregnancy, you can experience bouts of insomnia as the aches, pains, and the baby's kicks can disturb your sleep. Having to go to the bathroom all the time doesn't help either.

So what can you do? There are several steps you can take to help your body cope with all its fatigue.

• Go to sleep earlier. Try to get at least eight hours of sleep a night.

• Take naps during the day. A short 15-minute catnap can really refresh you.

• Eat healthy mini-meals throughout your day. This can keep your energy reserves up and prevent that sluggish feeling due to inadequate nutrition.

• Eliminate junk food from your diet. These foods can increase your fatigue.

• Keep hydrated with plenty of fluids. Dehydration can exhaust you.

• Exercise every day. Believe it or not, exercising will keep your energy levels higher during pregnancy and it helps prepare your body for labor.

• If you work, you may want to cut back your hours. If you can, take a day off in the middle of the week to build up your energy.

Because fatigue is a normal symptom of pregnancy, it is not something to worry about.

{Tip} If you feel that you are excessively tired, you may want to talk to your doctor. It is possible that your fatigue stems from low levels of iron in your blood.

COMPLICATIONS DURING PREGNANCY

Abnormal Pap Smear

At your first prenatal visit (at week 8), you should have undergone a pelvic exam, which should include a pap smear. During a pap smear, also called a pap test, cells are collected from your cervix and they are examined for signs of infection, cancer, or other conditions that could lead to cancer. When something seems off, the results are called "abnormal."

In women who have regular pap smears, abnormal changes are always caught early. If you get an abnormal pap smear, you will need further testing and possibly a biopsy of the involved tissue to find out what's going on.

If the abnormal cells show a sign of an infection, you should be treated and your pregnancy will continue on normally. Sometimes an abnormal pap smear shows pre-cancerous cells. There are various grades of severity – mild, moderate, or severe – and they will determine your course of treatment.

The main cause of an abnormal pap smear is a HPV (human papillomavirus) infection – a common sexually transmitted disease that causes genital warts and has been linked to cancer of the vagina, vulva, and cervix. In some women, your immune system clears the virus quickly so the infection goes away on its own. This is not the case in other women. Some women with a HPV infection do not show any symptoms until genital warts appear during their pregnancy. HPV infections can be treated with medications and creams during pregnancy without harm to your baby.

{Fact} An HPV vaccine is now available to protect against two types of HPV that cause cervical cancer. It is not recommend for pregnant women, but it is safe for moms who are breastfeeding.

Choriocarcinoma

Choriocarcinoma is a severe form of gestational trophoblastic disease (GTD) discussed in Week 5's chapter. GTD is a group of rare tumors that occur due to an abnormal growth of cells inside a woman's uterus. Unlike cervical cancer or endometrial cancer, GTD starts in the cells that would normally develop into the baby's placenta during pregnancy.

In most cases, choriocarcinoma is diagnosed after the cells that have been part of a normal pregnancy or a molar pregnancy (which was discussed in detail in Week 5) become cancerous and have spread to other parts of the body. This cancer can grow very quickly and cause symptoms within a short period of time.

Vaginal bleeding that continues after delivery can be a sign of this cancer. But persistent bleeding is most often due to retained placental tissue after delivery.

Choriocarcinoma is extremely rare and only happens in 1 of every 50,000 to 100,000 pregnancies. You can develop this cancer months or even years after you were pregnant. In over half of the cases, it occurs after a molar pregnancy. In other cases, it can happen after any type of pregnancy, including pregnancies that resulted in a healthy baby, miscarriages, ectopic pregnancies, and abortions.

Chemotherapy (cancer drugs) is the main type of treatment for choriocarcinoma. In rare cases, radiation therapy and a hysterectomy may be needed.

In patients whose cancer has not spread, they can be easily cured and it doesn't harm their chances of getting pregnant again. When the choriocarcinoma has spread to other areas, such as the liver or the brain, it may be harder to cure. However, around 70 percent of the women who initially have a poor outlook will go into remission.

Older women over age 35 and Asians have a higher risk of developing choriocarcinoma. If you have had a complete molar pregnancy in the past, you have a 15 percent chance of developing another GTD or choriocarcinoma.

{**Fact**} Choriocarcinoma can give you a false positive pregnancy test, because it produces high levels of the pregnancy hormone, human Chorionic Gonadotrophin (hCG).

WEEK
10

You have reached the end of your embryonic period!

Letter from Dr. James Brann •

This week marks the end of your embryonic period. From this point onward, your baby is at a decreased risk for physical birth defects, which often occur during the first nine weeks of pregnancy. Remember he/she is not out of the water for other birth defects, including chromosomal and genetic defects.

In my own practice, week 10 is usually the time that I refer my older patients (those over 35) and those at higher risk for genetic disorders to see genetic counselors. Because genetic defects tend to increase with age, this is something older women may want to pay careful attention to. We will cover genetic disorders and genetic testing in detail in this chapter.

Remember to continue healthy eating and lifestyle habits, and avoid harmful pollutants to ensure your baby continues to develop normally.

This is also the week that I receive phone calls from my patients concerned about bleeding gums and other dental issues. Is this normal? (You will discover the answer in this chapter).

As you may recall, your baby was starting to develop sex organs last week (week 9). By Week 10, the male babies are already producing and releasing testosterone!

Best Wishes,

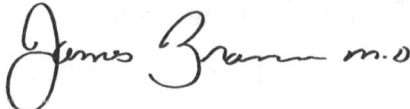

FETAL DEVELOPMENT

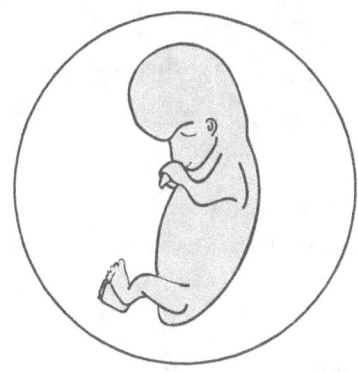

Congratulations! Your little one is no longer considered an embryo! Week 10 marks the end of the embryonic period. From conception until now, your baby has grown from a single cell to nearly 1 billion cells that make up your growing baby's anatomic structure. In the next few weeks, more growth and organ maturation will take place. At this point, your baby is at a lower risk for congenital malformations (birth defects), which normally occur during the first nine weeks.

Although you have made it to 10 weeks, keep in mind that exposure to pollutants, such as secondhand smoke, can have adverse effects on your growing baby. If possible, continue to avoid situations that can put you in contact with these pollutants.

Your baby is now 1.22 inches long and weighs about .14 ounce! He or she is a little larger than a lime.

Slightly decreased from last week, your little one's heart is beating 169.03 per minute with a running total of 7,409,125 heartbeats in his/her short lifetime.

By 10 weeks, your baby's brain makes up almost half of his/her total body weight!

Even though there is no air in your womb, your baby can display intermittent breathing motions now.

Your unborn baby can pee! His/her kidneys can now produce urine and will release it into the amniotic fluid.

In the developing male babies, his developing testes have already begun to produce and release testosterone.

This week, your baby's outer skin is no longer completely transparent! It is developing into a multi-layered membrane and will soon be losing a majority of its transparency.

Your little one's eyebrows are beginning to grow, and hair is appearing around his/her mouth!

By week 10, your baby's bones, joints, muscles, nerves, and the blood vessels of his/her limbs closely resemble that of an adult.

{Fact} Believe it or not, but right or left-handedness is developing! 75 percent of babies show right-hand dominance at this stage of development. The other 25 percent are either left-handed or show no preference.

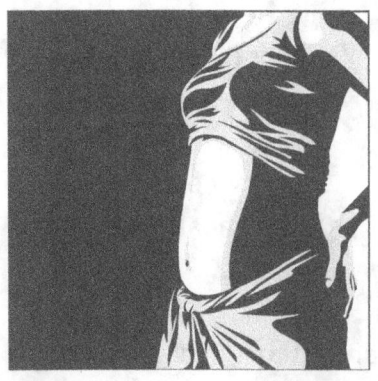

MOM'S PREGNANY SYMPTOMS

Hang in there! Now that you're 10 weeks pregnant, you only have a couple more weeks to go before you get some significant relief from your morning sickness. Your nausea and vomiting may be reducing in frequency around this week. You might already feel a bit better.

In the next few weeks, your body will change much more rapidly. You're probably feeling very pregnant now, even if no one else is the wiser. Your husband or partner may also start to notice some changes in your shape before too long. If you want to document the progression of your pregnancy, this is a great week to start. Around week 10, many women begin to keep a photographic record of their belly to show its change from week to week.

By this week, some women may have already heard their baby's heartbeat for the first time at the doctor's office, although most women have to wait a couple more weeks. Many first-time mothers describe the sound of their baby's heartbeat like the sound of galloping horses. If you have not already scheduled for your prenatal visits, you should do it as soon as possible.

Your breasts are continuing to grow this week, and you may also begin to notice some changes in your gums, including swollen gums and bleeding when you brush. Although a regular part of pregnancy, you want to make sure you maintain your regular daily dental care.

PREGNANCY 411

Birth Defects

Worried about birth defects? You are not alone. Most pregnant women want to deliver a healthy baby with no health or physical problems. In most cases, your newborn will be healthy. Only two or three newborns out of 100 babies have birth defects. Also called a congenital disorder or malformation, a birth defect is a physical problem that can be recognized right away at birth or later in the baby's life. Birth defects can be mild or severe, and they can affect how the child's body looks and functions.

{Fact} Older women (over age 35) are at an increased risk of delivering a baby with a birth defect. The risk of birth defects continues to increase with age.

Some birth defects can be prevented by avoidance of harmful things, such as chemicals and medications, during pregnancy. In other cases, birth defects are inherited as a result of genes or chromosomal problems. In about 70 percent of birth defects, the cause of the defect is not known.

Some babies with birth defects can be treated with surgery or medication. Most birth defects occur within the first three months of your pregnancy. Some can be detected with special screening tests. The results of these special tests, along with genetic counseling, can provide parents with their risk factor for having a baby with birth defects.

{Fact} Heart defects are the most common type of birth defect, affecting about 1 in 125 newborns.

Genetic Disorders

Birth defects that are inherited are called genetic disorders. To understand genetic disorders, it's important to understand the basics of genetics:

• A man's sperm and a woman's egg each carry 23 chromosomes. When they join together in the fertilization process, the 23 chromosomes from the sperm and the 23 chromosomes from the egg pair up to give the fertilized egg 46 total chromosomes. The fertilized egg then develops into your baby.

• One set of chromosomes from the woman's egg and the man's sperm are called sex chromosomes. These determine whether your baby will become a boy or a girl. Your egg always carries a female chromosome (X). The sperm can carry either an X or a Y (male) chromosome. So, the baby always gets an X chromosome from you, and either an X or Y chromosome from the father. A combination of XY sex chromosomes will create a boy, and XX chromosomes create a girl.

• Chromosomes are made up of many different genes. When the chromosomes pair up to create your baby, genes also pair up. You pass specific traits, such as eye and hair color, to your baby through genes. Genes can be dominant or recessive. Dominant genes work alone to influence your baby's characteristics. In a gene pair, dominant genes will cancel out instructions given by recessive genes. For a recessive gene to show up in your baby, both genes in the pair must be recessive.

• Like with eye or hair color, genetic disorders can be passed to your child through genes. They can be caused by problems with either the entire chromosome or with the genes in the chromosome.

When a gene is passed from parent to child, it's called an inherited disorder. There are three types of inherited disorders: dominant, recessive and X-Linked.

• **Dominant disorder:** One parent carries the dominant gene for a disorder or disease. The child's chance of getting the disorder is one in two (50 percent). Examples of dominant disorders include polydactyly (your baby has extra fingers or toes).

• **Recessive disorder:** Both parents must carry the recessive gene before it can affect their child. Everyone carries a few abnormal recessive genes. Most of the time, they don't cause any problems because the normal genes will override the abnormal gene. If you are a carrier (you carry the recessive gene for a specific disorder), you may not have any signs of the disorder but you can pass it to your children. If both parents are carriers, the child has a 25 percent chance of having the disorder. If only one parent is a carrier and the other isn't, the child will also be a carrier. Examples of recessive disorders include cystic fibrosis, sickle-cell disease, and Tay-Sachs disease.

• **X-Linked Disorder:** Also called "sex linked" disorders, these are caused by an abnormal gene on the X (female) chromosome. Because many x-linked disorders are due to a recessive gene, they tend to affect boys more frequently than girls. Females have an extra X chromosome to cancel out the abnormal one, so x-linked disorders rarely affect girls. Boys have a Y chromosome that does not cancel out the abnormal X chromosome, so they will inherit the disorder. If the father is normal and the mother is a carrier, the child has a 50 percent chance of inheriting the disorder. Only if the mother is a carrier and the father has the disease will the daughter inherit the disease. Examples of these disorders include hemophilia and fragile X syndrome.

{Fact} A birth defect can also be caused when a parent passes a normal chromosome to the baby, but this chromosome changes or mutates later. This is called a non-inherited disorder.

Common genetic disorders include:

• **Sickle Cell Anemia -** A serious blood disorder in which your body makes abnormally shaped (crescent-like) red blood cells. Normal red blood cells are circular or disc-shaped, and they can move through your blood vessels with great ease. Sickle cells (the crescent ones) do not move easily through your blood vessels, often forming clumps and getting stuck in the vessels. These blocked blood vessels can cause severe pain, serious infections, and organ damage. Sickle cell anemia affects 1 in 600 African-American babies and 1 in 1000 Hispanic babies. Millions of people worldwide have the disease. Although there is no universal cure, a small number of people have been helped with bone marrow transplants. Doctors are continuing to improve treatment and care for this disorder.

•**Tay-Sachs Disease -** A rare disorder that destroys nerve cells in the child's brain and spinal cord. It can cause mental retardation, blindness, and seizures. Babies with this disorder appear normal until they reach 3 to 6 months old. At this time, their development slows down and their muscles weaken. They also have seizures, vision loss, hearing loss, and paralysis. A common sign of the disease is a cherry-red spot inside the back wall of their eye that can be identified by a doctor. Because there is no cure for the disorder, children with Tay-Sachs Disease usually die by age 4 or 5. Although rare in the general population, it is more common in people of eastern and central European Jewish heritage (Ashkenazi Jews) and French Canadians.

•**Cystic Fibrosis -** A disorder that affects the child's lung and digestive system. It can cause problems with breathing. It affects about 30,000 children and adults in the United States each year. A defective gene causes you to create a thick and sticky mucus that clogs the lungs and obstructs the pancreas. This obstruction stops the pancreatic natural enzymes that help your body break down and absorb food. People with the disease often have a persistent cough, frequent lung infections, shortness of breath, and poor weight gain despite a good appetite. Over 70 percent of cystic fibrosis patients are diagnosed before they are two years old. About one in 2,500 Ashkenazi Jewish babies are born with the disease each year. There is currently no cure, and the median age of survival is 37 years.

•**Thalassemia** - A blood disorder that makes your blood produce fewer healthy red blood cells and less hemoglobin (the iron-rich protein in your red blood cells that carries oxygen to other parts of the body). This genetic disorder causes mild or severe anemia – a condition that can cause fatigue along with a number of other symptoms, including shortness of breath, chest pain, dizziness, cold hands and feet, and pale skin. There are varying degrees of disease severity. In some cases, blood transfusions may be needed throughout the person's life. The most severe type can lead to infant death shortly before or after birth. Thalassemia affects both boys and girls, and it occurs most often among Italians, Greeks, Middle Eastern people, Asians, and those of African descent.

•**Hemophilia** - A rare x-lined genetic disorder in which your blood doesn't clot normally. After a cut or injury, you may bleed for a longer period of time than people without the disease. If you have an accident and bleed internally, this can become life threatening. People with hemophilia have little or no blood proteins that help them form blood clots. Without these blood proteins, you will not stop bleeding. Although there is no cure for this disease, hemophilia patients can get injections of blood clotting factors to stop bleeding. About 400 babies are born with the disorder annually. It only occurs in boys (with a few rare occasions in girls).

{**Fun Fact**} Queen Victoria of England was a carrier for hemophilia, and she passed it on to many of her descendents.

Chromosomal Disorders

Birth defects can also be the result of chromosomal disorders – such as a missing, damaged, or extra chromosome. These are rarely passed from parent to child. They normally occur when the egg and sperm join at the time of conception. Children with chromosomal disorders can face severe health problems, including physical and mental defects.

Your risk of giving birth to a baby with a chromosomal disorder increases as you get older. A 35-year-old woman has a 1 in 192 chance of having a baby with one of these disorders, but her chance increases to 1 in 66 when she reaches 40-years-old.

Common chromosomal disorders include:

• **Down Syndrome** - Also called Trisomy 21, this is a common chromosomal condition. Instead of having the 46 total chromosomes (which is the normal number), Down Syndrome babies have an extra chromosome for a total of 47 chromosomes. This additional genetic material can led to a combination of birth defects, including mental retardation, abnormal facial features, heart defects, hearing problems, and vision disorders. The severity of their disorder can range from mild to severe. People with Down Syndrome can lead fulfilling lives. Some even attend college and get married. Although there is no treatment for the disorder, life expectancy is around 60 years old. The disorder affects 1 in every 733 births. Over 400,000 people in the U.S. have Down Syndrome.

• **Trisomy 18** - This is a chromosomal condition in which the baby has an extra copy of chromosome 18. This disorder can cause severe mental retardation and physical abnormalities, including a heart defect and open spinal column. Because of the life-threatening medical problems that come with the disorder, most babies will die within the first month of life. Only 5 to 10 percent live past their first year. Trisomy 18 affects 1 in every 3,000 newborns. It affects mostly girls (80 percent).

• **XXY or Klinefelter's Syndrome** - This condition affects boys who have an extra chromosome, the female X chromosome. Instead of the regular XY chromosome pattern, these boys have an XXY pattern. As babies, they have weaker muscles so they learn how to sit up, crawl, and walk later than normal babies. When they reach adolescence, they do not produce as much testosterone as normal boys, so they tend to have larger breasts, round hips, weaker bones, and lower energy levels than other boys. Between 95 to 99 percent are infertile. About one of every 500 to 1,000 male babies are affected by this disorder.

• **Turner Syndrome** - This disorder only affects girls. Instead of having two X chromosomes, these girls have a missing or incomplete X chromosome. As a result, these children are shorter, start puberty late, and are often infertile. Their ovaries often do not work properly. They are at higher risk for high blood pressure, kidney problems, cataracts, thyroid problems, diabetes, and osteoporosis. Turner Syndrome affects 1 in 2,500 girls. Although there is no cure, growth hormones can help them grow taller, hormone replacement treatment can stimulate their sexual development, and assisted reproduction techniques can help some get pregnant.

Multifactorial Disorders

Birth defects can also be caused by the combination of genetics and environmental factors. These are called multifactorial disorders. Some of these disorders can be detected during pregnancy, and they can often be treated with surgery. Examples include cleft palate, clubfoot, and neural tube defects (such as spina bifida).

• **Cleft Palate** - This occurs when there is a split in the baby's upper lip and roof of the mouth. As a result, many children with cleft palates have a gap between the nose and the mouth. Surgery can close the gap and make the child's face appear more normal. This birth defect is very common, affecting 1 or 2 out of every 1,000 babies born in the US. Although we do not know why some babies develop this birth defect, it may be due to lack of sufficient vitamins during pregnancy, exposure to cigarette smoke, medication or drugs the mother may have taken during pregnancy, and possibly genetics.

• **Clubfoot** - When a baby is born with clubfoot, his/her foot is bent abnormally inwards. Sometimes, it looks like the baby's foot is upside down.

The joints and tendons on the inside and back of the child's foot and ankle are shorter than they should be, while those on the outside and front are stretched out. Without treatment, it can be painful to walk. Close to 50 percent of the babies with clubfoot have two affected feet. Although the cause is not known, it may be due to genetics. Most of these children are otherwise healthy, but some do face other neurological and chromosomal conditions. Treatment includes a series of corrective casts and surgery. One out of every 1,000 babies has clubfoot.

> {**Fun Fact**} Famous British poet, Lord Bryon was born with club-foot. Other famous people with the disorder include figure skater, Kristi Yamaguchi and football player, Troy Aikman.

• **Spina Bifida** - A neural tube defect (a problem that affects the spinal cord and its covering) that develops in the first trimester when the baby's spinal column doesn't close all the way. Often, children with spina bifida need braces, crutches, and wheelchairs for support. No one knows what causes spina bifida, but it's suggested that a combination of genetics, nutritional deficiency (especially lack of enough folic acid in the mom's diet during pregnancy), medications taken during pregnancy, diabetes, and obesity can increase the risk of the disorder. Treatment includes surgery, physical therapy, and medications to help manage the complications. It affects 1,500 newborns annually.

> {**Tip**} Taking folic acid can prevent neural tube defects, such as spina bifida. For it to be effective, you should take it daily before your pregnancy and throughout the first three months.

Screening for Birth Defects

Although you cannot prevent all birth defects, understanding your risk factors can help you make the right decisions about your pregnancy. Women who are over 35, have a family history of birth defects, have another child with a birth defect, are taking certain medications when they become pregnant, or abuse illegal drugs or alcohol are at higher risk of giving birth to a baby with a birth defect.

If you are at higher risk, genetic counseling and testing can be done before, during, and after your pregnancy. Remember that birth defects can also occur even when there is no family history of it.

A variety of tests are used to check for birth defects. These include carrier testing, prenatal screening tests, and diagnostic testing.

Carrier Testing

Some birth defects can be inherited from you or your partner. Carrier testing is performed to see if a couple carries a gene for inherited disorders. These include cystic fibrosis, sickle cell anemia, Tay-Sachs disease, and thalassemia. If carrier tests are performed before you get pregnant, you can decide if you want to get pregnant or not.

In a carrier test, a sample of your blood or saliva is studied to detect any abnormal genes that can pass to your baby. If your test result shows you are a carrier for a specific disorder, the next step is to test your partner or the baby's father. If the test shows that both parents are carriers, a genetic counselor can give you more information on your risk of passing it to your child.

Prenatal Screening Tests

During pregnancy, prenatal screening tests can be performed to look for signs that your baby might have a genetic defect. The results of these tests only show if there is an increased risk that a defect will occur, not if your baby has one.

Common problems found through screening tests include neural tube defects, Down syndrome, and trisomy 18.

Screening tests are easy to perform and will not harm your baby. You can choose a single test or a combination of them. Your doctor should explain the risks and benefits of the screening tests to help you make good decisions.

In the first trimester, screening tests include blood tests and a special ultrasound exam. These can be done between 11 and 14 weeks of pregnancy to detect your baby's risk for Down syndrome and trisomy 18.

A special ultrasound exam, called nuchal translucency screening, can be performed in the first trimester to measure the thickness at the back of the baby's neck. An increase in thickness can signal a genetic defect.

The combination of blood tests and nuchal translucency screening can detect Down syndrome in many cases (82 to 87 percent).

In your second trimester, a blood test called "multiple marker screening" is used to test for Down syndrome, trisomy 18, and neural tube defects. This test measures the levels of certain hormones and proteins in your blood to determine the risk of certain disorders.

> {**Fact**} **When first and second trimester tests are used together, they can predict Down syndrome in 90 to 95 percent of cases.**

Diagnostic Testing

If a screening test raises concern about the baby's health, diagnostic testing can be used to find out if your baby has certain disorders. These tests can include amniocentesis, chorionic villus sampling, and fetal blood sampling.

An amniocentesis is usually performed between 15 and 20 weeks of pregnancy. During this procedure, the doctor guides a thin, hollow needle through your abdomen and uterus to collect a sample of the baby's amniotic fluid. The amniotic fluid is sent to a lab, where cells from the baby that were shed in the amniotic fluid are grown into a special culture. These cells are then studied under a microscope. When the results come back, you will know if your baby has any chromosomal defects from the study of those cells. From the chemistry of the amniotic fluid, you will know if your baby has any neural tube defects or other problems.

Common perception is that an amniocentesis will cause you a lot of pain, but in reality, you will most likely feel a pinch or a needle stick and pressure. Although amniocentesis is safe for the most part, complications can arise. Side effects can include vaginal bleeding, cramping, leaking amniotic fluid, and infection. There is also a small chance of miscarriage (0.5 percent risk).

{Fact} An early amniocentesis can be done, before 15 weeks, but it poses a higher risk of miscarriage.

Another diagnostic test, chorionic villus sampling (CVS) also detects the same chromosomal problems as an amniocentesis, but it can be performed earlier. Often, you can get the CVS procedure at 10 to 12 weeks of pregnancy. During a CVS test, the doctor will take a small sample of cells from your placenta, where the placenta attaches to the wall of your uterus. These cells, called chorionic villi cells, were formed from the fertilized egg, so they have the same genetic makeup as the baby.

There are two methods for a CVS procedure. The doctor may guide a small tube through your vagina and cervix to collect the cells (transcervical), or he can collect the cells by inserting a needle through your abdomen and uterus and into your placenta (transabdominal).

After the sample is collected, it is sent to a lab where the cells will be grown into a culture, so the chromosomes can be studied for chromosomal and other genetic defects. Because the CVS procedure does not test amniotic fluid, it does not test for neural tube defects.

{Fact} If you have Rh-negative blood, after a CVS procedure, your physician will give you an injection of RhoGAM to prevent Rh sensitization – a condition in which your Rh-negative blood makes antibodies that will attack the Rh-positive blood cells of your baby.

Like with amniocentesis, CVS comes with some risks. Infections can occur, and in rare cases, limb deformities in babies have occurred when the procedure occurred before 9 weeks. There is about a 1 percent chance of a miscarriage.

When the results of amniocentesis and CVS are unclear, fetal blood can be used to test for chromosomal defects, blood disorders, and other abnormalities. In fetal blood sampling, also called cordocentesis, a needle is inserted in the mother's abdomen and blood is taken from a vein in the baby's umbilical cord. This test is only used between week 18 and week 22 of pregnancy.

Like with other diagnostic tests, there are potential side effects to fetal blood sampling, such as blood loss from the puncture site, infection, premature rupture of membranes, and the baby's heart rate dropping. Miscarriage can also occur, but there is a 1 to 2 percent risk.

NORMAL CHANGES TO EXPECT

Breast Changes

When you are pregnant, your breasts undergo remarkable change as your body gets ready for breastfeeding. Early on, you may have noticed that your breasts felt swollen, tender, and tingly. By 6 weeks, they may have even grown an entire bra cup size!

Expect your breasts to continue to grow in size and weight for the first three months of your pregnancy. You may even experience discomfort and pain as this happens. This is due to the fat layer of your breasts thickening and the number of milk glands increasing.

During pregnancy, your heart has to work harder to pump more blood to the womb, so it can support your growing baby. As your blood flow increases, you may see bluish veins that appear underneath the skin of your breasts. Don't be surprised if your nipples and the pink or brownish skin around them (called areolas) darken. Many pregnant women also report that their nipples begin to stick out more, and their areolas grow larger.

The glands on the surface of your areolas (called Montgomery's tubercles) may also rise up and become bumpy. During pregnancy, these tiny bumps secrete an oily substance that lubricates your nipples and aerolas.

> {Tip} If you have flat or inverted nipples (nipples that stick inward toward the breast), breastfeeding may be difficult. You should talk to your doctor or a breastfeeding specialist about your concern early in your pregnancy.

As your breasts get bigger, they can be very tender and sensitive to touch. Don't be surprised if each of your breasts increase by 2 inches or up to 3 pounds during pregnancy.

By the end of your first trimester, you may notice that your breasts have started to leak a thick yellow fluid, called colostrum. Don't be alarmed! This leakage is normal and it just shows that your breasts are preparing to produce milk. Colostrum may leak by itself or dribble when your breasts are massaged or when you are sexually aroused.

Although yellow at first, colostrum will become pale and almost colorless as your birth draws closer. For a few days after birth, colostrum will nourish your newborn until your breasts start to produce regular milk. Colostrum is not only rich in fat and calories, but it also contains water, minerals, proteins, and antibodies that will protect your child from disease.

If your breasts don't leak during your pregnancy, this shouldn't worry you either. Not all women experience leakage. This will not affect your ability to breastfeed.

> {Fact} As your breasts grow in size and weight, they might feel itchy and you might develop stretch marks. Some women's stretch marks will start to fade after their baby is born.

Gum and Tooth Changes

Your mouth is not immune to the havoc that your pregnancy hormones can create. The shift in your hormones increases the blood flow to your gums and can cause them to become more sensitive and irritated. As a result, your gums may swell or bleed after you brush your teeth. You also become more susceptible to gingivitis during pregnancy. If you have pre-existing gingivitis, it can worsen when you are pregnant.

Gum changes can start to appear around the end of your first trimester, or after the second month of pregnancy. Your gums will go back to normal after you deliver your baby.

{Tip} To lessen your gum irritation, switch to a softer brush.

To prevent gingivitis and other gum disease during pregnancy, it is very important that you continue to practice good oral health, including brushing and flossing your teeth on a regular basis. Don't skip your regular dental checkups just because you are pregnant.

The increased level of pregnancy hormones in your body can also change how your body responds to bacteria. This can make it easier for plaque to build up in your mouth, leading to cavities and other dental problems.

If you can, schedule a dental checkup early in your pregnancy to ensure that your mouth continues to stay healthy. Delaying dental work can lead to more problems. Several studies have linked gum disease to pre-term labors and low birth weights.

If you need dental work, always let the dentist know that you are pregnant. Local anesthesia and dental X-rays won't harm your baby as long as they are done with the baby's safety in mind. It's important to wear abdominal shields if you get an X-ray to avoid being exposed to unnecessary radiation.

Pregnancy tumors, which are non-cancerous inflammatory growths that develop on your gums, can also occur during pregnancy. They are usually painless, but they should be treated. These tumors are caused by your body's inflammatory response being extra sensitive to local irritants, like plaque, during pregnancy.

> {**Fact**} Pregnancy tumors are rare, and they only occur in 0.05 to 5 percent of all pregnant women.

COMPLICATIONS DURING PREGNANCY

Inflammatory Bowel Disease

Inflammatory bowel disease (IBD) is the name for a group of conditions that cause your digestive tract, including the intestines, to become inflamed (red and swollen). The inflammation can last a long time and cause abdominal cramps, pain, diarrhea, weight loss, and intestinal bleeding. There are two major types of IBD: Crohn's disease and ulcerative colitis (UC).

Researchers don't know what causes IBD, but they think that genetics, environment, and diet can play a role. Like with other illnesses, stress can make the symptoms of IBD worse.

Women who struggle with inflammatory bowel disease often worry about how their IBD will affect their fertility and the baby's health during pregnancy. In most cases, the disease doesn't hurt a woman's ability to get pregnant. However, extensive surgery to treat IBD can increase infertility because of the scar tissue that results from the surgeries.

If you have IBD, the extent of your disease will impact your symptoms and your baby's health during pregnancy. Women with more severe disease-during pregnancy have a higher risk for delivering early and having a low birth weight baby.

Women with active disease are more likely to suffer from their symptoms when they are pregnant and their symptoms may also get worse. On the other hand, two-thirds of the women who are in remission when they first get pregnant continue to stay in remission throughout their pregnancy. When relapse occurs, it often occurs during the first trimester.

Doctors recommend that IBD patients wait until they are in remission before they try to get pregnant.

Because of the genetic component of inflammatory bowel disease, your baby is at increased risk of developing the disease. First-degree relatives, such as siblings and children, of people with IBD have a 3 to 20 percent chance of developing the disease.

{Fact} Over 600,000 Americans have some type of inflammatory bowel disease. Between 15 and 30 percent of IBD patients have a relative with the disease.

Inflammatory bowel disease is often treated with medication. Because some medications can increase the risk of birth defects, be sure to talk to your doctor about the medications you are taking.

{Fact} There has been no evidence that IBD will get worse because of breastfeeding. All women are encouraged to breastfeed as it is beneficial to both baby and mom.

Anemia During Pregnancy

When you are pregnant, your blood vessels expand as your blood volume increases. Because the volume of your blood is increasing so rapidly, the concentration of your red blood cells can become diluted and cause you to become anemic. This can decrease the amount of oxygen available to the baby, and this can lead to poor fetal growth, miscarriage, premature births, and low birth weights. That's why it is important to prevent anemia during your pregnancy.

Pregnant women are usually tested twice for anemia – during your first prenatal visit and then at 28 weeks when you are screened for gestational diabetes.

Anemia occurs when you don't have enough healthy red blood cells in your body. You may experience fatigue, lack of energy, irregular heartbeat, dizziness, pale skin, and shortness of breath.

Iron deficiencies are the main cause of pregnancy-related anemia. Most women often do not have the iron stores required to handle the nutritional demands of their growing baby. As a result, they can become anemic and need additional iron supplements. Iron is normally prescribed as part of a prenatal multivitamin or as a separate supplement.

If your doctor prescribes iron, remember to take it with food to avoid nausea. Avoid taking it with milk; the calcium will prevent the iron from being absorbed into your body. Instead, take your iron pill with orange juice or another form of vitamin C. Vitamin C helps absorption.

{**Fact**} **Between 16 and 29 percent of pregnant women experience anemia in their third trimester. Anemia tends to be the worst at the end of the second trimester and beginning of the third trimester.**

In the cases of severe iron deficiencies, after other treatments have failed, a red blood cell transfusion might be needed.

When you are pregnant, remember to eat iron-rich foods and sources of vitamin C to avoid anemia. Iron-rich foods include red meats, eggs, leafy green vegetables (such as spinach and broccoli), dried beans and tofu, and dried fruits (such as raisins, prunes, and apricots).

An iron deficiency can also go hand-in-hand with a folic acid deficiency. Folic acid is a B-vitamin that works with iron to make new cells, including red blood cells. It's very important to get enough folic acid in your diet during pregnancy.

You can find folic acid in whole wheat products, fortified breakfast cereals, meats, beans, asparagus, leafy green vegetables, and fruits (such as oranges, strawberries, and melons).

Thalassemia and sickle cell anemia (see the "Pregnancy 411" section of this chapter) can cause anemia.

Three weeks to go until your second trimester!

Letter from Dr. James Brann •

You only have three more weeks to go before you reach your second trimester. I hope this is an exciting time for you and your family. Your morning sickness and fatigue should be steadily decreasing by now, and soon you will feel much better.

You may still have mixed emotions about your pregnancy. It's absolutely normal to feel emotional, and even shedding a tear or two can be healthy for you. Near the end of their first trimester, many of my patients find themselves tuning into parenting and health channels that focus on pregnancy. Learn as much as you can from these TV shows and this book, so you can have a successful rest of your pregnancy.

By week 11, you may notice that your waist and hips are expanding. Maybe your old clothes no longer fit. It's often fun to start looking at maternity apparel. There are many options out there, and I wish you the best of luck in finding a stylish pregnancy wardrobe.

If fall or winter is upon you, you may worry about getting sick. When it starts to get cold, my office is always bombarded with phone calls about the safety of the flu vaccine and the possible dangers of the flu on pregnant women. I

will discuss this topic in detail under the "Complications During Pregnancy" section of this chapter.

Your baby is starting to grow his or her teeth this week! Although these "teeth" are only tiny buds right now, this is still an exciting development!

Best Wishes,

James Brann m.o.

FETAL DEVELOPMENT

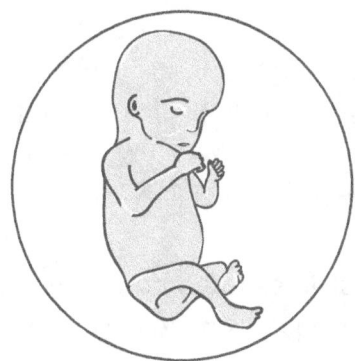

Your little baby is growing strong. By week 11, he/she has over 90 percent of the same structures as an adult! Your little one is now big enough to be held in the palm of your hand and measures 1.61 inches from crown to rump. Your baby now weighs in at 0.25 of an ounce!

Your little baby's heart rate now averages 168.06 beats per minute. Throughout his/her total lifetime, the heart has beat 9,103,216 times!

You will be amazed at all the actions your baby can perform at this early stage of development. By now, your baby can swallow amniotic fluid, suck his/her thumb, grasp objects, move his/her head backwards and forwards, close and open his/her jaw, move his/her tongue, sigh and stretch. The list goes on and on.

By now, tiny buds have sprouted in your baby's mouth. These buds will eventually grow into teeth!

Vocal ligaments have started to appear in the baby's larynx, which signals the beginnings of vocal cord development.

Your little one's external genitalia are still forming, but they are distinguishable. Your baby is now either a girl or a boy! Because it is so early in the pregnancy, an ultrasound will not yet be able to detect the sex of your baby. You must wait until week 18 to find out!

In the female babies, the uterus can be identified. Immature reproductive cells, called "oogonia," are replicating in your little girl's ovary.

> {**Fact**} Between week 11 and week 12, your baby will have a huge burst of growth. By next week, your little one will have increased his/her body weight by over 75 percent!

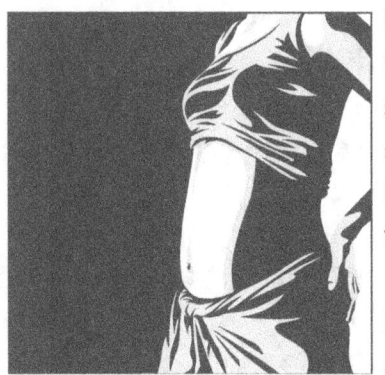

MOM'S PREGNANCY SYMPTOMS

Hip, hip hooray! You are finally starting to show this week! Though you still won't be showing a lot (especially if this is your first baby), other people may begin to notice that you are pregnant.

If your morning sickness has not already abated by now, it should completely disappear pretty soon (for most women, anyway). By week 11, many women also notice a decrease in their fatigue. Their energy levels are slowly coming back as they head into the "honeymoon" period of pregnancy – the second trimester!

As your second trimester approaches, your risk of miscarriage significantly drops. Most miscarriages occur in the first 13 weeks of pregnancy.

> {**Fact**} Around week 11, your uterus is thinking about sticking out your pelvic bone. When this happens, you will start to appear even more pregnant.

Some women also experience intermittent cramping in their first trimester. This cramping tends to be mild and is located along the lower part of your abdomen. It is common but it should not be persistent and increase in severity.

PREGNANCY 411

Large Family Size

The size of your family is a very personal decision that both you and your partner should make early in your pregnancy. If you want a large family, there are some things you must consider, including your age and physical health.

When making the decision about your family size, you should take into consideration:

• **Your lifestyle** - Does your family or career take priority in your life? If you are career-oriented, do you have a supportive partner or the ability to hire good and reliable childcare? How much time and energy do you have to devote to your children? Just one child or several?

• **Personal and religious beliefs** - What are your beliefs and ideologies when it comes to birth control and family planning?

• **Financial Situation** - Children are expensive. The U.S. Department of Agriculture estimates that a middle-income two-parent family will spend over $220,000 on raising a child from birth until their high school graduation. Can you afford to raise more than one child? Are you willing to sacrifice other luxuries to have more children?

There are advantages and disadvantages of both a larger family and a smaller one, and this is something you should think over carefully.

If you are an older woman (over 35) who wants to have many children, you may find that as you get older, you face an increased risk of pregnancy complications.

Grand multiparity is the medical term for women who have had five or more pregnancies. The number of pregnancies can include fetal deaths (babies that die in the womb after 20 weeks of pregnancy) and stillborns (babies born without a heartbeat).

Grand multiparous mothers are at a higher risk for placenta previa (your placenta grows in the lowest part of your uterus, and this can cause severe vaginal bleeding) and placental abruption (your placenta detaches from your uterus wall, which may cause vaginal bleeding and can pose a danger to your baby).

Younger grand multiparous mothers (under 35) are at lower risk compared to older mothers with the same number of children. It is very possible that the increased risk of these complications may be related to the mother's age. (We covered maternal age and how it relates to pregnancy in Week 8.)

{**Fact**} You are at higher risk for complications with your first pregnancy, but this risk decreases after your first baby is born. Your risk will not increase again until your fifth pregnancy.

Back-to-Back Pregnancies

During pregnancy, your body is constantly working to support your growing baby. Everything gets thrown out of whack—from your abdominal muscles to your breasts. After you've delivered your bundle of joy, your body must recover and heal from your pregnancy, labor, and delivery.

Recovery doesn't happen overnight. It may take time before your body goes back to normal and your nutritional stores are replaced. That is one of the reasons that many doctors recommend that you wait at least two years before you get pregnant again.

However, accidents do sometimes happen and you can become pregnant again without planning to. In some cases, women may want to have children close in age. Although having a planned back-to-back pregnancy is a personal choice, you should be aware of the risks involved.

Since pregnancy and breastfeeding can zap up many of the nutrients in your body, having a second baby while you are breastfeeding can be tough on your still-recovering body. As a result, your body may not be able to support and nurture your new baby as easily as it did the first.

Babies conceived less than 6 months after you gave birth can raise your risk for certain pregnancy complications, including preterm births and low birth weight babies.

These pregnancy complications may be due to your body not having enough time to restore your nutritional reserves. Postpartum stress may also play a role.

> {**Fact**} Stress during pregnancy can sometimes increase your heart rate and blood pressure, and neither of these is good for your developing baby.

If you do not want to become pregnant again, it is important to use some form of birth control when you have sex. Mothers who are not nursing can become fertile again a few weeks after delivering. If you are breastfeeding, it can be difficult to tell when you ovulate.

Breastfeeding should not be used as a temporary method of birth control. Although nursing can prevent ovulation (the release of the eggs from your ovaries), it is only effective under certain circumstances:

• Your baby is six months or younger. After six months, you are at higher risk of pregnancy if you do not use another method of birth control.

• You must breastfeed constantly. In order to suppress your ovulation hormones, you must breastfeed as often as your baby needs it. Do not let four hours in the day, and six hours at night, pass without breastfeeding.

• You are exclusively breastfeeding. Your baby should not get his or her nutrition from any other source but your breast milk. (No formula or solid foods).

• Your period has not returned yet.

When all these circumstances are met, breastfeeding is 98 percent effective. However, if you do not want to get pregnant again, you should supplement breastfeeding with another form of birth control (such as spermicides or condoms).

Once your baby starts nursing less, sleeping for longer periods of time, and eating solid foods, this breastfeeding method of birth control will no longer be effective.

{Fact} Although there is no "right" gap to become pregnant again, your risk for preterm births, small baby size, and low birth weight also increases if it has been five years since you last gave birth.

NORMAL CHANGES TO EXPECT

Waistline and Hip Expansion

In the next six months, expect your pregnant body to continue to expand as it works to nurture your developing baby. This is partly due to your growing uterus and the increase level of hormones in your body.

Throughout your pregnancy, your body produces a hormone called relaxin. In the first trimester, relaxin helps with the implantation and growth of your placenta. Later in your pregnancy, this hormone prepares your body for the labor and delivery process. It allows the ligaments in your hip to stretch, which causes your hip bones to separate and makes your hips wider.

Relaxin also relaxes your symphysis pubis (a pubic bone located in the middle front part of your pelvis) and softens your cervix to get your body ready for the baby's birth.

At the same time that your hips are widening, your uterus will expand to make room for your little one, and this will cause your abdominal muscles to stretch. The buildup of fat, water retention, and increase of gas in your bowel will also make your waistline bigger.

Hip and waistline expansion are a normal part of pregnancy, but they can affect your musculoskeletal system – the muscles and bones that move your body. It can lead to uncomfortable pregnancy side effects, including back pain, pelvic pain, and hip pain.

If you experience back pain or hip discomfort during this expansion process, you can ease your pain through various methods:

• Wear low-heeled (but not flat) shoes that have good arch support.

• Sit in chairs that have good back support, or place a small pillow on your back for extra support.

• Sleep on your side with pillows between your knees for support. A good pregnancy pillow is a great option.

• Apply heat, cold, or massage to the area of your body that hurts.

Clothes Getting Too Tight

As your hip and waistline expand during pregnancy, you will notice that your regular clothes begin to feel tight. By week 11 of your pregnancy, you may have already noticed this.

{**Fact**} **Many of today's hip and modern moms-to-be embrace their growing bellies and choose not to hide behind maternity clothes. You may want to opt to wear larger sizes in regular, everyday wear!**

If you are like other women, you may worry that wearing tight clothes could hurt your growing baby. Perhaps you've heard the rumor that wearing tight clothes constricts your blood flow, so your baby does not receive the amount of oxygen that he or she needs. Some pregnant moms even claim that tight clothes cause their heartburn, varicose veins, and light-headedness to become worse. Don't worry! These are all rumors. Although wearing tight clothes may be uncomfortable for you, it will not hurt your baby in any way. Your little one is growing safely under layers and layers of muscles and skin, in addition to being protected by amniotic fluid, the placenta, and your uterus.

When your jeans begin to get too tight, you can opt to buy a maternity belt (also called belly belts). These attach to your regular jeans or pants and stretch to expand the waistline. This is an inexpensive alternative to buying maternity clothes. They are ideal for moms on lower budgets who need a quick fix to their expanding body.

If you want, you can purchase maternity apparel to accommodate your size. These clothes tend to be elastic and loose, and they conform to your growing body. They come in a variety of styles and fashions.

When buying maternity clothes, remember that they should always be comfortable. Never buy clothes that restrict your arms, legs, or feet. If you are carrying twins or multiples, you may have a harder time finding maternity clothes in your size. In these cases, you may want to check out specialty shops online that cater to your needs.

{Fact} As your breasts become larger during pregnancy, you may want to invest in a comfortable maternity bra. These will ease some of the heaviness and pain that you may have.

COMPLICATIONS DURING PREGNANCY

Normal Seasonal Flu

When you're pregnant, your immune system changes and this can make you vulnerable to common illnesses and diseases.

In a non-pregnant woman, common illnesses, such as the cold or flu, can be easily treated with over-the-counter medications and prescriptions. However, when you are pregnant, these medications may cause harm to your growing baby. As a result, doctors have special considerations to make when it comes to treating pregnant women.

Influenza (also called "the flu") is a common illness that pregnant women must pay special attention to. The flu is a very contagious viral respiratory infection that is spread from person-to-person. Symptoms of the flu include high fever, extreme tiredness, coughing, sore throat, runny or stuffy nose, muscle aches, and fever.

Pregnant women face more flu-related complications, such as pneumonia and dehydration, than non-pregnant women. These complications can cause severe illness, hospitalization, and even death.

In the average flu season, it is estimated that 25 out of 10,000 pregnant women in their third trimester will require hospitalization for flu-related complications. These complications can be even more severe if the expectant mother has a pre-existing illness, such as asthma, diabetes, and heart disease.

The increased risk for flu-related complications may be due to the change in your immune system during pregnancy, your heart working harder than before to support your growing baby, and pregnancy predisposing you to pulmonary edema (fluid building up in your lungs).

> {Fact} Between 5 and 20 percent of the U.S. population catch the flu annually. On average, over 200,000 people are hospitalized from flu-related complications, and around 36,000 people die each year.

It is not well understood how the flu virus will affect your baby's health. There has been little evidence that it increases your risk for birth defects, still births, or premature births. Although there have been a few studies that the influenza virus can affect the baby through the placenta, this is very rare.

> {Fact} Pregnant women with pneumonia tend to have preterm labor and deliveries and low birth weight babies.

Pregnant women who are infected with the flu are treated with rest, fluids, and Tylenol. They are often monitored closely for serious complications that may arise. Antibiotics may be needed for flu-related pneumonia, sinus infections, and ear infections. Treating the flu with antiviral medications (such as Tamiflu) is not recommended because it may increase the risk of birth defects.

During pregnancy, it is very important to try to prevent the flu. If you're going to be pregnant during the flu season (October – March), you should get a flu vaccine. A flu shot will protect you for at least six months. Because the flu shot does not have live virus, it is considered safe at any stage of pregnancy. However, you may experience some fatigue and muscle aches after the flu shot, but this is just your immune system responding to the vaccine.

The nasal flu mist is not approved for use in pregnant women.

You can also prevent the flu by practicing good hygiene. You should wash your hands often, avoid large crowds, avoid contact with people who are sick, and do not touch your eyes, nose, or mouth.

Call your doctor immediately if you have trouble breathing or if your symptoms don't get any better.

{Tip} If you get sick, do not take any over-the-counter medications or herbal products without consulting your doctor first.

H1N1 ("Swine") Flu

Pregnant women are in the high-risk group for developing complications from the H1N1 flu (sometimes called the "swine flu"). Even healthy pregnant women with no pre-existing illnesses are at higher risk than regular people.

Like with the seasonal flu, changes in your immune system, lungs, and heart can make you prone to illness from this new strain of the influenza virus. The H1N1 virus spreads in the same way that the regular flu is spread, but it has caused more severe illness and even death in pregnant women.

More pregnant women die from the H1N1 flu as compared to the general population. This is why it is important for pregnant women to get vaccinated.

Symptoms of the H1N1 flu virus include fever, cough, sore throat, runny or stuffy nose, headache, chills, fatigue, and body aches. Some people also experience vomiting and diarrhea.

You may be concerned with the safety of the H1N1 flu vaccine. This vaccine is produced in the same way as the regular flu vaccine, which has been given to millions of pregnant women for over 45 years. The mercury in the H1N1 flu vaccine will not harm you or your child. There has been weak evidence linking thimerosal (the mercury in the vaccine) to autism. However, if you are still concerned, in some areas of the country, you can get a H1N1 flu shot that does not include mercury.

You have a higher risk of getting sick with the H1N1 flu without the vaccine than with it.

In extremely rare cases (1 out of 1 million people), the H1N1 flu vaccine may cause Guillain-Barré Syndrome (GBS – a disorder in which your immune system damages its own nerve cells, and it can cause muscle weakness and sometimes paralysis). If you have ever had GBS, it is important to tell the person giving you your flu vaccine.

> {**Fact**} **Fevers can be dangerous to your unborn child. Tylenol is often recommended for pregnant women to lower their fevers.**

Women with the H1N1 flu are at higher risk for premature deliveries. In past swine flu pandemics, pregnant women with the flu had higher risks for miscarriages and stillbirths. Therefore, it is very important for you to be treated for the flu immediately after the onset of symptoms.

WEEK 12

Ready to hear your baby's heartbeart?

Letter from Dr. James Brann •

What an exciting week you have ahead of you! Week 12 is often the first time that you will hear your baby's heartbeat! You will be in awe when you hear how vibrant and alive your little one is. It will fill you with love and pure joy.

As your second trimester fast approaches, you may have relief from your morning sickness, but get ready for the back aches, lower abdominal discomfort, and round ligament pain that you will begin to experience. These are just some "joys" of pregnancy that you have to look forward to.

We will discuss round ligament pain under the "Changes to Expect" section of this chapter.

Remember to continue healthy eating habits and good hygiene to prevent sickness. In this chapter, we will also discuss two common viruses that are not well known, but can cause great harm to your baby if you are exposed to them during pregnancy: toxoplasmosis and cytomegalovirus.

Best Wishes,

James Brann m.d.

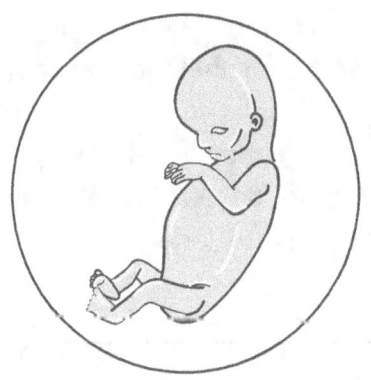

FETAL DEVELOPMENT

What an exciting time it is for your baby. Since last week, he or she has had a significant growth spurt. Your little one is not so tiny anymore! He or she now weighs around 0.49 ounce and measures 2.13 inches long from crown to rump!

Your baby's heart rate is now averaging about 167.10 beats per minute.

By now, he/she is very active. To pass the time, your baby is yawning, sucking his/ her thumb, and opening and closing his/her mouth.

If stimulated, your baby can roll his/her eye downward.

Most of the bones in your little baby's body are continuing to harden. His/her fingernails and toenails are beginning to develop this week.

Although you may not be able to feel your baby move inside you for several more weeks, he/she is constantly moving.

{Fact} When you look at an ultrasound of your baby at week 12, you will be amazed at all the intricate details of your baby's body that you can see, including his/her little feet and hands.

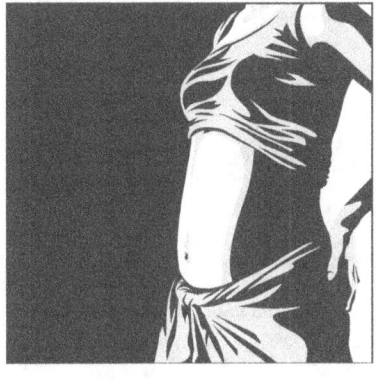

MOM'S PREGNANCY SYMPTOMS

If you weren't showing yet last week, this may be your week! Week 12 is often the time when many women realize that their uterus has risen above their pubic bone and pelvis. When this happens, it creates a small pooch in your lower abdomen and makes you look pregnant.

Around 12 weeks, you may notice that your skin pigmentation changes. You may begin to develop chloasma – dark splotches that form on your face. Also called "the mask of pregnancy," chloasma is very common in pregnancy and is caused by the rising levels of pregnancy hormones in your body. Sun exposure can increase your risk for developing this skin condition. Luckily, these dark splotches will begin to fade away after your baby is born.

{Fact} **Chloasma affects between 50 – 70% of all pregnant women!**

You may also notice other skin changes on your body. If you haven't already noticed little bumps developing around your nipples or areolas, you may start to see them now. These bumps are called "Montgomery's tubercles," and they are an almost universal pregnancy symptom caused by your pregnancy hormones.

Although your nausea and morning sickness should be improving, you may notice that your heartburn and indigestion are becoming increasingly worse. As your baby grows larger and the uterus moves up into your abdomen, it will place pressure on your intestines and contribute to heartburn and indigestion problems. This will not go away until after your baby is born. (You can read more about heartburn and indigestion in Week 8's chapter under "Changes to Expect During Pregnancy.")

{Tip} **Now that you are appearing more pregnant, you may have a beautiful "pregnancy glow" about you. This may be a great week to announce your pregnancy to the world!**

PREGNANCY 411

X-Rays

X-rays are necessary for doctors and other healthcare professionals to make diagnoses. If you have a serious fall or accident, or if you need dental work, you may be asked to have an x-ray. Under normal circumstances, this would not be a problem. However, when you are pregnant, having diagnostic x-rays and other medical radiation procedures can concern you.

Although it is rare that you will need an x-ray during pregnancy, it is always important to understand your risks of potentially harming your growing baby. X-rays have varying degrees of harm, depending on the location of your body being x-rayed and the amount of radiation that you are exposed to.

If properly performed, x-ray examinations on your arms, legs, head, chest, or teeth will not directly expose your uterus or growing baby to radiation, so these are considered safe. However, x-rays that target your lower torso – such as abdomen, stomach, kidneys, pelvis, and lower back – may expose your baby to the direct x-ray beam, and they need special considerations.

> {Tip} If you need an x-ray, excluding those in your abdomen and lower torso, be sure to wear a lead chest guard to minimize the radiation that you are exposed to.

Researchers disagree on whether the small amount of radiation used in x-rays and other diagnostic radiation procedures can actually harm your baby, but they do agree that your developing baby is highly sensitive to external agents.

Your unborn baby is most sensitive to radiation in the first 14 days after conception. The further along you are in your pregnancy, the less damage radiation will do to your unborn child.

Although low doses of radiation are considered safe during pregnancy, it is always best to avoid getting x-rays if possible. High doses of radiation can increase your risk of miscarriage and increase your child's chance for mental retardation, stunted growth, birth defects, and cancer later in life.

Studies have linked certain childhood cancers, particularly leukemia, to exposure to low levels of radiation during pregnancy.

> **{Fact}** If you have been exposed to less than 5 rads of radiation, there is no evidence that you are at an increased risk of birth defects, mental disability in your child, small babies, or miscarriage. But there may be a small increased risk of childhood leukemia (one in 2,000 children versus the regular rate of 1 in 3000 children). Keep in mind that a regular chest x-ray is only 0.001 rads.

Don't be alarmed if you have to get an x-ray during pregnancy. Even if you need an abdominal x-ray, the risk to your baby is very small. As with anything else, you should weigh the benefit of finding out about your medical condition against the risk to your baby.

Because diagnostic x-rays can provide your doctor with important, and sometimes life-saving, information about your medical condition, they should be used if you have no other options.

If an abdominal x-ray is needed, you can reduce your risk of exposure by telling your doctor that you are pregnant. He may be able to postpone the x-ray or reduce the amount of radiation you receive.

Sex During Pregnancy

If you are having a normal, low-risk pregnancy, you can continue to have sex with your husband or partner. You can continue to have sex safely up until you deliver, unless your doctor or healthcare professional has warned you against it.

Having sex will not harm your baby in any way, and it will not cause preterm labor or deliveries. Your baby is protected inside your amniotic sac, and your cervix protects your little one from germs.

> **{Fun Fact}** The contractions that you may feel during and after an orgasm are different from the ones you will feel in labor.

However, just because sex is safe during pregnancy, this doesn't mean you will have a desire for it. During your first trimester, your morning sickness and fatigue may put a damper on your sex drive. In the latter part of your pregnancy, your huge belly might make sex uncomfortable.

Some pregnant women report that sex feels different than before. Some may find it more pleasurable; others may not. When you are pregnant, the increase in your blood flow may cause your genitals to swell up, which can heighten your sensations or it could make you uncomfortable. Some women also experience cramps during and immediately after sex. If the cramps don't go away after a few minutes, or if you have bleeding after sex, call your doctor.

Although sex is generally safe during pregnancy, it is not recommended for high risk pregnancies or for women who are experiencing certain complications, such as threatened miscarriage, preterm labor, placenta previa (your placenta is situated at the opening of the uterus), unexplained vaginal bleeding, and discharge of your amniotic fluid.

Always have open and honest communication with your partner about sex. Talk about other ways to be intimate, including kissing, cuddling, fondling, mutual masturbation, and oral sex. You may want to experiment with different positions to find the one that is most comfortable to you.

NORMAL CHANGES TO EXPECT

Round Ligament Pain

As your uterus continues to expand and you grow larger, you may begin to experience a dull ache or sharp pain on one side of your abdomen. This is called "round ligament pain," and it is a very common pregnancy experience. Although these pains can occur at the end of your first trimester, they are most common between 18 and 24 weeks.

When your pregnancy began, your uterus was the size of an apple or a pear. As your baby grows inside you, the ligaments (bands of strong tissue) that support your uterus on both sides begin to stretch. When these ligaments, called "round ligaments," stretch, they pull at nearby nerves and other sensitive structures, giving you pain in your lower belly and pain that radiates into the groin.

More women experience round ligament pain on their right side rather than their left. However, some pregnant women experience pain on both sides. Any movement (even every day ones, like changing positions, coughing, or laughing) that quickly stretches these ligaments can trigger pain.

{Tip} If you experience round ligament pain, bend toward it to relieve the pain. If you can, avoid changing positions too quickly. Moving more slowly will allow your round ligaments to stretch slower, minimizing the pain you feel.

Any kind of pain during pregnancy can cause you to worry, but round ligament pain is normal and should only last between a few seconds to a few minutes. This pain tends to be a sudden onset of sharp pain that becomes a dull ache with time. It should go away with rest.

If your pain is more severe or doesn't go away, you should call your doctor. If you experience fever, chills, bleeding, cramping, nausea and vomiting, or changes in your vaginal discharge, contact your doctor immediately. This may be a sign of something more serious. In some cases, pregnant women have confused round ligament pain with more severe problems, including appendicitis and ovarian cysts.

Round ligament pain may last through your second and third trimesters as well. Once your baby is born, this pain can be an intermittent problem until your uterus returns to its normal size (about six to eight weeks after delivery).

{Tip} If your round ligament pain becomes too unbearable, you can talk to your doctor about what pain medications are safe to take.

Nosebleeds & Nasal Congestion

Although seeing blood gush out of your nose can be a frightening experience, don't worry if this happens to you. Nosebleeds are a very common pregnancy experience. The increase in your hormones and the extra blood supply in your pregnant body can change the mucus membranes inside your nose and cause them to swell up, dry out, or bleed easily.

Like the other blood vessels in your body, the ones in your nose expand and become more delicate during pregnancy. This will cause them to burst easily.

You are more likely to have a nosebleed when you have a cold, sinus infection, or allergies. Dry environments, such as airline cabins and cold weather, can also lead to nosebleeds. Although they are messy and inconvenient, nosebleeds are common and pretty harmless during pregnancy.

{Fact} Around 60 percent of adults have experienced a nosebleed in their lifetime. Only 10 percent of these require medical attention.

When you have a nosebleed, remember to stay calm. You can stop a nosebleed with these tips:

• Always keep your head higher than your heart.

• Press your thumb firmly against the side of the nostril. Apply pressure for five to ten minutes. Don't let up for a second, even if you think the bleeding has stopped!

• Remember to breathe normally.

• Lean forward slightly to prevent blood from running down your throat. You can either sit or stand still. Do not lie down or tilt your head back.

• After five to ten minutes, release the pressure gradually.

Applying ice may help stop a nosebleed too. You can hold an ice pack or a bag of frozen veggies over your nose and cheeks with your free hand. Ice can help constrict your blood vessels.

> {Tip} Once your bleeding has stopped, be careful not to do anything that may flare it up, such as blowing your nose or bending over.

Along with nosebleeds, the changes in your nose's mucus membranes can also give you a stuffy or runny nose.

To ease any nasal discomfort and to prevent runny noses and nosebleeds, you may want to:

• Use a humidifier to keep the air in your home moist.

• Drink plenty of water and liquids to keep your nasal passages moist.

• Apply a bit of petroleum jelly around the edges of your nostrils. This will keep the skin moist.

• To relieve congestion, try saline drops or spray. Always let your doctor know what over-the-counter decongestants, nose drops, and nasal sprays you want to use beforehand.

• If you have to blow your nose, blow it gently. Blowing your nose too hard can give you nosebleeds.

• When you sneeze, keep your mouth open.

> {Tip} If you experience nosebleeds too often, let your doctor know.

COMPLICATIONS DURING PREGNANCY

Toxoplasmosis
Toxoplasmosis is a common parasitic infection that affects over 60 million

people in the U.S. every year. Most people who carry the disease have very few symptoms because their immune system keeps the parasite dormant and prevents it from causing illness. When symptoms are present, they tend to be mild and flu-like, such as swollen glands, fatigue, muscle aches, and fever.

You can get toxoplasmosis from handling cat litter that is infected with the parasite. You can also become infected by eating uncooked meat from animals that were infected or by consuming food that came into contact with contaminated meat.

Active infection only occurs once in your life. Once you are infected, the parasite lies dormant (inactive) in your neural and muscle tissue for the rest of your life. However, you will have built an immunity against it, so it will not cause any side effects or harm unless you have a compromised immune system (such as AIDS).

Toxoplasmosis can have disastrous effects on your baby if you are exposed to the parasite for the first time during pregnancy. If transmitted to your baby, he or she is said to have congenital toxoplasmosis. This parasitic infection can damage your child's eyes, nervous system, and ears. Your baby may also face blindness, severe mental retardation, and neurological problems later in life. Babies who are exposed to toxoplasmosis in the first trimester face the most severe consequences.

A majority of infected babies do not have any symptoms present at birth, but they will develop them later in life. If signs are present at birth, they may include fever, swollen lymph nodes, jaundice, an usually large or small head, anemia, and an enlarged liver or spleen. Infected babies are treated immediately after birth to prevent long-term problems.

Luckily, women who developed immunity to the parasite before they became pregnant will not pass it to their baby.

Doctors recommend that women with new toxoplasmosis infections wait at least six month before getting pregnant.

> **{Tip}** If you want to know whether you currently have toxoplasmosis or have been infected in the past, your doctor can test you with special blood tests.

If you are pregnant and get toxoplasmosis, don't fret. Certain medications and antibiotics are used to treat the infection. Prevention, however, is key to protecting your unborn child's safety.

To prevent toxoplasmosis:

• Be sure to cook meat thoroughly. Use a food thermometer as an extra precaution. Your meat should not be pink; the juices should be clear.

• Wash all cutting boards, utensils, dishes, sink, and counters that have been in contact with raw or undercooked meat with hot, soapy water.

• Always thoroughly wash all fruits and vegetables.

• Avoid drinking unfiltered water.

• If you are pregnant, avoid traveling to underdeveloped countries, especially South America, where stronger strains of the parasite exist.

• Avoid changing your cat's litter box. If you cannot avoid this chore, always wear gloves and wash your hands thoroughly afterwards.

• Wash your hands with soap and water after cooking or gardening.

• When you garden, always wear waterproof gloves.

Cytomegalovirus (CMV)

Similar to toxoplasmosis, cytomegalovirus (CMV) is a very common virus that is passed from person-to-person and can infect people of all ages. CMV is a member of the herpes virus family, and once it gets into your body, it stays there for life. But in a person with a healthy immune system, the virus stays dormant or silent, producing few or no symptoms at all. Like with toxoplasmosis, if you do develop symptoms, they tend to be mild and flu-like. These symptoms may include severe tiredness, headache, high fever, chills, and an enlarged spleen.

Between 50 to 80 percent of American adults will be infected by CMV by the time they are 40 years old. Children are normally infected in early childhood, especially if they attend childcare or preschool. Because most people have no symptoms, you may never know that you've been exposed to CMV unless you are tested for the virus.

CMV can cause serious problems for people with weakened immune systems and for the unborn babies of infected women. Because it can be passed from the infected mother to her baby during pregnancy, birth, and breastfeeding, it is a virus to pay special attention to. CMV is the most common virus transmitted from mother to child during pregnancy.

Like other common viruses, CMV can be spread through close contact with an infected person. Healthcare and lab workers, moms of young children in childcare, and childcare workers are at high risk of getting CMV. In the infected person, the virus can be passed through bodily fluids, including blood, saliva, semen, cervical secretions, breast milk, and urine.

Pregnant women commonly contract a CMV infection through sexual contact with an infected person. They can also get the virus through contact with the saliva or urine of young children who have been infected.

One to four percent of pregnant women will experience their first CMV infection during pregnancy. About one-third of these women will pass it on to their child. Minorities and people with lower household incomes have higher rates of infection.

If you have already been infected with the virus before pregnancy, you have less than a 1 percent chance of infecting your child.

Most babies born with CMV will never develop any symptoms or disabilities. Some babies may have temporary symptoms that go away in time. These may include jaundice (yellow skin), liver problems, purple skin splotches, low birth weight, and spleen problems.

In other cases, the damage from the virus can be permanent and leave these children with serious disabilities, such as hearing or vision loss, mental disability, small head size, lack of coordination, seizures, and even death.

In the United States, 1 in 150 babies are born with a CMV infection, but only 1 in 750 children will develop serious disabilities from it. Every year, close to 8,000 children suffer from permanent disabilities as a result of CMV.

An estimated 10 percent of CMV-infected infants will have symptoms at birth, but the other 90 percent show no symptoms. Out of these 90 percent, between 10 to 15 percent will develop symptoms months and sometimes years after birth.

{Fact} Although CMV is not as well known as other viruses and diseases, more children have serious disabilities due to CMV than other well-known conditions, such as Down syndrome, spina bifida, pediatric HIV/AIDS, and fetal alcohol syndrome.

If you are worried that your baby was born with CMV, your doctor can test his or her urine, saliva, and blood for the virus. This must be done within the first three weeks after birth. Luckily, babies that become infected with CMV after birth are not at risk for any disabilities.

Because there are no safe and effective drugs to treat CMV in pregnant women, prevention is key:

- Wash your hands frequently with soap and water for at least 15 to 20 seconds.

- Avoid contact with people who are sick.

- Do not kiss young child under the age of 5 on the mouth or cheek. Kiss them on the head instead.

- Do not share food, drink, and utensils with young children.

- If you work in a childcare center, you can reduce your risk of catching CMV by working with children who are older than two.

- Avoid sexual contact with multiple partners.

PRENATAL CARE

Fetal Heartbeat

Congratulations! You have made it to 12 weeks and your second prenatal visit. What an exciting time this must be for your family. At this visit, your doctor will be checking your weight, blood pressure, and urine (for protein and sugars in the urine). He will also feel the top of your uterus to make sure your baby is still growing and developing normally. The most exciting part of this visit is that you will be able to hear your baby's heartbeat for the first time!

For the last 12 weeks, your baby's heart has been growing strong. By now, your baby's heart is fully developed, but his or her autonomic nervous system (which regulates the baby's heartbeat) is continuing to develop. The autonomic nervous system is part of your central nervous system and also helps regulate your lungs, intestines, stomach, and various other functions.

As you read under this week's "Fetal Development" section, your baby's heart rate now averages about 167.10 beats per minute. This is pretty fast! But as your little one continues to grow, his or her heartbeat will slow down. The reason for this is the imbalance in the autonomic nervous system early in pregnancy.

The autonomic nervous system regulates your baby's heartbeat (also called fetal heart rate), and it works through a balance of two components – the sympathetic nervous system (which regulates your "fight or flight" response and increases your heart rate and blood pressure when it senses "danger" or a threat) and the parasympathetic nervous system (which calms your heartbeat and decreases your blood pressure, allowing you to sit back and relax).

Right now, the sympathetic nervous system has more control over your baby's heartbeat, but as the weeks pass, the parasympathetic nervous system will begin to neutralize and balance its partner out. As a result, your baby's heartbeat will begin to slow down. For example, at week 20 of your pregnancy, the average fetal heart rate is 155 beats per minute, and at week 30, it will decrease to an average of 144 beats per minute.

{**Fact**} A normal fetal heart rate is between 110 and 160 beats per minute. A heartbeat not in that range may signal a problem.

During your second prenatal visit at week 12, your doctor will use a Doppler ultrasound to listen to your baby's heartbeat. This is a small, hand-held device that is placed on your belly, and uses sound waves to calculate your baby's heartbeat.

A majority of the time, your doctor will be successful in finding your baby's heartbeat. But because your little one's heart is still very tiny, it may be difficult to find in some circumstances. Don't freak out if this happens. Your doctor can elect to do a transvaginal ultrasound to verify that your baby is still alive and has a heartbeat.

During a transvaginal ultrasound, the transducer (the handheld device that sends and receives ultrasound signals) is inserted into your vagina, instead of sitting on your belly. Because your baby is still small at 12 weeks, transvaginal ultrasounds produce a better image and more accurate reading of your baby's heartbeat. Remember to empty your bladder before a transvaginal ultrasound!

WEEK

13

Say Goodbye to the First Trimester!

Letter from Dr. James Brann • • • • • • • • • • • • • • • • • • •

It's the last week of your first trimester! This is an extremely exciting time for my patients as their morning sickness and fatigue is finally winding down. Most start to experience relief from their other pregnancy symptoms. The second trimester is often called the "honeymoon" of pregnancy, so you should look forward to it!

If you are like my patients, you may be worried about what medications are safe to take during pregnancy. Although I would advise you to try to stay away from any drugs or medications during pregnancy, because no medicine is 100 percent safe, you must weigh and balance the risk versus the benefit of the medicine that you take.

In this chapter, I have compiled a list of over-the-counter medicines to treat common ailments that are considered "safe" to take when you are expecting. Always talk to your healthcare provider and doctor before taking any drugs – whether over-the-counter or prescription.

Continue to take good care of yourself. Avoid being around sick individuals and maintain healthy hygiene.

Best Wishes,

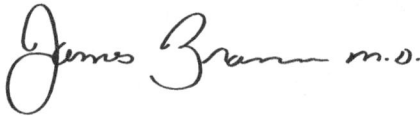

FETAL DEVELOPMENT

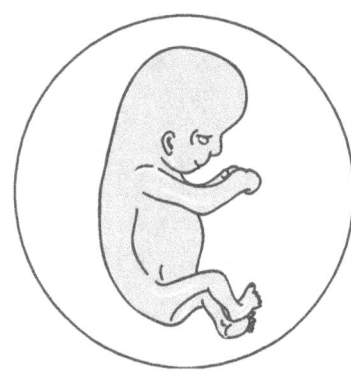

Your baby is growing very quickly! This week, he or she is continuing to gain weight and grow in length. Over the next week, your baby will have increased his or her weight by nearly 60 percent.

At 13 weeks, your little one has grown to about 2.91 inches and weighs 0.81 ounce!

Your little one's intestines are moving to their permanent resting place.

The intestines are beginning to absorb glucose and water from the amniotic fluid that your baby has been swallowing.

Your baby's pancreas has started to produce insulin – which helps regulate blood sugar levels later in life.

By now, your baby's nose and lips are completely formed, and they will continue to change their appearance as your baby continues to develop.

MOM'S PREGNANCY SYMPTOMS

If you haven't already experienced the "ouch" of round ligament pain, you will soon know what it is! As the ligaments (bands of strong connective tissue) in your lower abdominal area stretch to support your grow-

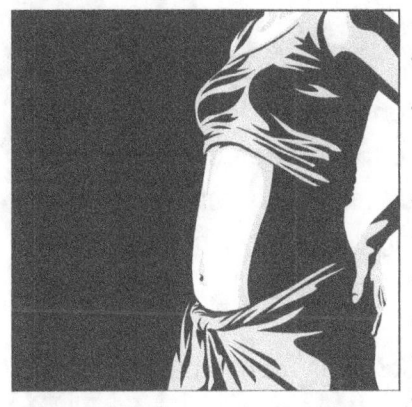

ing uterus, you may feel a sharp pain on the side of your belly. Don't be alarmed – this is a typical pregnancy change!

Although round ligament pain is more common in the second trimester, women do experience this pain in the latter part of their first trimester. To relieve the pain, you may want to rest and take your time when moving from one position to the next. (We discussed round ligament pain in detail in Week 12.)

You may not look too big at week 13, but as you enter your second trimester, you will begin to pack on the pounds! Your baby is going to need more fuel to grow and develop, so don't be surprised if you start to eat more. In the second trimester (which starts next week), women of average weight start to gain close to a pound every week. This may also be due to the fact that your morning sickness should be completely gone by now, and your appetite is finally returning.

As you continue through your pregnancy, acne may become a problem. The increase of hormones in your body may cause you to break out more when you are pregnant. This is normal, even if it's unpleasant for you. You can treat your pimples by washing your face with mild cleansers several times a day. Be careful of some acne products as they may contain chemicals that cause birth defects.

> {Tip} During pregnancy, doctors do not recommend using accutane (isotretinoin) or tetracycline to treat your acne. Accutane can cause major birth defects (both internal and external), miscarriage, premature births, and mental retardation in surviving babies. Tetracycline can cause fetal harm and permanent discoloration of the baby's teeth.

PREGNANCY 411

Medications During Pregnancy

During pregnancy, medicine can cross the placenta and enter your baby's blood stream. While some medications are perfectly safe to take and won't harm your baby, others can lead to birth defects, miscarriage, stillbirths, and reduced fetal growth. They may also impair or halt the development of important organs, including your baby's central nervous system.

Medicine, both over-the-counter and prescription, can impact your baby at different stages of his or her development. They may be more dangerous in the beginning of the pregnancy, but safer closer to your due date. If you are on prescription medication, your doctor may take you off your regular medicine and put you on another medication that is safer for your unborn baby.

{Tip} Do not stop taking your prescriptions just because you are pregnant. Always talk to your doctor or healthcare provider about what medications are safe to use during pregnancy.

The FDA (U.S. Food and Drug Administration) requires that all drugs list their risks for pregnant women and women trying to get pregnant. Before you take any new medications, read the warning labels carefully. Your doctor, nurse, and pharmacist can assist you in finding medications that are safe to take during pregnancy.

If you are on prescription medication, you should weigh the risk of taking your medication against the effect of not taking them. For example, some diseases are more harmful to your baby than the drugs used to treat them.

You may want to stay away from herbal products, minerals, amino acids, and other "natural" products during pregnancy. These have not been proven safe for pregnant women and women who are nursing. You may want to ask your doctor or healthcare provider about taking these.

Because no medication is 100 percent safe, it is always best to stay away from taking medicine when you are pregnant, unless it is absolutely necessary.

{Fact} You have to pay special attention to the medicines you take during your first trimester, as this is a very critical time of your baby's development. Some medications are only safe to take in the second trimester.

SAFE OVER-THE-COUNTER MEDICATIONS DURING PREGNANCY

ALLERGIES

Saline Irrigation	Rinsing your nose with a saline solution can be more effective than a saline spray, as it uses a larger amount of water. This technique rinses out the allergens and irritants from your nose to treat drainage, nasal dryness, and congestion. It can be used before applying nasal sprays for a better result. Saline irrigation kits are available over-the-counter.
Cromolyn Sodium Nasal Sprays (NasalCrom)	These over-the-counter medicated nasal sprays treat runny noses and chronic asthma, but it may take 2 to 4 weeks before you see results. It's approved for pregnancy because only a small amount of the drug is absorbed into your blood stream.
Antihistamines	These are available over the counter, and they relieve your itchiness, sneezing, and runny nose. They do not help nasal congestion, so they are often used with decongestants. Only a few antihistamines are safe during pregnancy: Claritin (loratadine), Zyrtec (cetirizine), and Benadryl (diphenhydramine).

Decongestants	Over-the-counter decongestants that are safe to use in pregnancy are Dimetapp and Sudafed. These are often used in conjunction with antihistamines. Use of these medicines after the first trimester has been linked to lower rates of premature birth, low birth weight babies, and fetal death, making doctors hypothesize that a runny nose in pregnancy may be a sign of good placental function. Decongestants should be avoided during your first trimester because not enough data is available to determine whether these drugs are safe to use or not. After the first trimester, you should only use it when you need it. Do not use these medicines if you have high blood pressure or preeclampsia.

{**Fact**} While these medications are basically safe in pregnancy, they may be excreted in breast milk. Always read the warning labels and talk to your physician first.

ACNE

Salicylic acid	Similar to aspirin, salicylic acid can be used in pregnancy but in smaller quantities. It is used to control acne, and it works to soften skin while destroying pimples. High doses in its oral form have been linked to birth defects and other pregnancy complications. (Read about the dangers of NSAIDs and aspirin in the next section). Salicylic acid is in many brand name acne medications, including Neutrogena, Stridex, and Dermarest.
Benzoyl peroxide	A commonly used ingredient in many acne medications, benzoyl peroxide can be used in pregnancy. It is often used in conjunction with clindamycin or erythromycin. Available over-the-counter and in prescription form, you can find this ingredient in gels, lotions, creams, masks, and acne cleansers.

| Benzoyl peroxide (continued) | Due to widespread use of topical antibiotics in acne, your body may have built up a resistance to these drugs (such as clindamycin and erythromycin), but combining these topical medications with benzoyl peroxide improves the effectiveness of these treatments. |

> {**Fact**} In pregnancy, acne can go in two directions. If you've had acne all your life, it can improve drastically. In contrast, women with no history of acne can develop horrible acne in pregnancy.

COLD & FLU

Tylenol (acetaminophen)	Acetaminophen is considered safe to use at all stages of pregnancy. For colds, it will relieve your sore throat, headaches, and fever. This drug is often the medication of choice that obstetricians recommend during pregnancy.
Saline Nasal Drops or Spray	This will also help relieve your runny nose. It is not medicated, so it's safe to use.
Air Humidifier	If you have a cold or flu, try using an air humidifier to help relieve your chest and nasal congestion.
Warm Salt Water Gargle	This is an effective way to relieve the discomfort of a sore throat.
Sudafed	A commonly used decongestant that is used in pregnancy.
Cough Suppressants	Robitussin DM, Vicks Cough Syrup, and Halls cough drops are safe to use during pregnancy.

CONSTIPATION

Bulk-Forming Fiber	These are considered the safest treatment for constipation during pregnancy since they are not absorbed into your blood stream. Over-the-counter

Bulk-Forming Fiber (continued)	products include: Metamucil, Fiberall, and Citrucil.
Docusate (Colace)	This stool softener can be used to treat constipation. It is safe to use when needed, but chronic use throughout pregnancy is not recommended.
Milk of Magnesia	Laxatives should be used with caution during pregnancy, as they may cause intestinal cramps. If used on a regular basis, they may make your intestines dependent on them. Milk of Magnesia is safe to use during pregnancy, but it is not a long-term solution. Only use it when you need it.
Senna (Senokot)	A natural laxative, Senna is considered safe in pregnancy. Like other laxatives, it should be used as a quick fix for constipation, not for long-term use.

> **{Fact}** To prevent constipation, drink more water and liquids and eat fiber-rich foods - such as fruits, vegetables, whole-grain bread, and beans.

DIARRHEA

Kaopectate	This is an anti-diarrhea that uses a clay-like substance. It is considered safe for use in pregnancy because the drug is not absorbed into your blood stream. However, it should only be used for 24 hours in the second and third trimesters.
Immodium	You can use immodium to treat acute diarrhea during pregnancy, but only after the first trimester. Do not use it for more than 24 hours.

FIRST-AID OINTMENTS

Neosporin	This commonly used ointment keeps germs away and occasional use is safe in pregnancy.
Bacitracin	Occasional use of this ointment will not harm your baby.
Polysporin	A Johnson & Johnson antibiotic ointment, Polysporin can be used when needed during pregnancy.

HEADACHE & PAIN RELIEF

Tylenol (acetaminophen)	When used for short periods of time, Tylenol is very safe and effective in treating headaches, aches, and pains during pregnancy.

{Fact} Aspirin is not recommended during pregnancy. The FDA warns against using it during the last three months of pregnancy because it can harm your baby and create complications during the labor and delivery process.

HEARTBURN

Anti-acids	This is the first line of relief for heartburn in pregnant women. Safe anti-acids include Maalox, Milk of Magnesia, Tums, Gaviscon, Titralac, and Mylanta.
Zantac (Ranitidine)	If anti-acids don't help your heartburn, you may choose to use Zantac. This is also safe and effective during pregnancy.
Riopan	This medication is also safe to use during pregnancy. It should be taken on an empty stomach.
Tagamet (Cimetidine)	This medicine is safe to use during pregnancy to treat heartburn, indigestion, and a sour stomach. Be sure to take it with food.

HEMORRHOIDS

Preparation H	This can be used safely in pregnancy to relieve hemorrhoids. Severe and recurrent hemorrhoids may require a special surgery, called hemorrhoidectomy, which can be safely performed in pregnancy.
Anusol (Hydrocortisone)	This can be used to treat hemorrhoids during pregnancy, but extensive use in large quantities or using for a long period of time is not recommended for pregnant women. You may want to stay away from hydrocortisone in your first trimester; some studies have linked using hydrocortisone in the first trimester to increasing your baby's risk of developing cleft palate and cleft lip.
Witch Hazel (Tucks)	Safe to use during pregnancy, witch hazel can help shrink hemorrhoids and can relieve the pain that comes with them.

MORNING SICKNESS

Ginger	Ginger and ginger-containing foods (like candied ginger or ginger lollipops) may help mild cases of nausea and vomiting.
Vitamin B6 (Pyridoxine)	This is a water-soluble B-complex vitamin that has very few side effects, and it is often the first line of defense against morning sickness.
Unisom (Doxylamine)	This sleep aid has been approved for use in pregnant women to help with morning sickness. It is often used in conjunction with vitamin B6.
Emetrol	This can be used to treat nausea that comes with morning sickness. However, it contains fructose, so diabetics should not take this medication.

Sea Bands	These are acupressure wristbands that are available over-the-counter and have become popular in recent years. These are perfectly safe to use during pregnancy.

RASHES & SKIN IRRITATION

Hydrocortisone Creams	These are safe to use during pregnancy for temporary relief of skin irritations, itching, and rashes. You should not use large quantities or use these regularly over a long period of time.
Caladryl Lotion (Praxoxine)	This medicine is used to temporarily relieve pain and itching from skin irritation and rashes. It is safe during pregnancy as long as you do not use it in large quantities.
Benadryl Cream (Diphenhydramine)	This is safe to use for pain and itching that comes with rashes. However, you should not use it during the first trimester of your pregnancy, as it may increase cleft palate formation. Higher doses of this medicine can be harmful during pregnancy.
Oatmeal Baths	These may provide relief of your rash or skin irritations during pregnancy. They are safe to use at any stage of pregnancy.
Calamine Lotion	This is perfectly safe to use to sooth your skin and provide relief when you need it.

YEAST INFECTION

Clotrimazole	Traditionally an anti-fungal medicine for athlete's feet, clotrimazole is also available to treat vaginal yeast infections. It is safe to use for relief of your symptoms.

Monistat (Miconazole)	A popular yeast infection medicine, you can continue to use this during pregnancy.

{Tip} When using medications to treat yeast infections, be careful not to insert the applicator too far because you may hit your cervix and start bleeding.

Non-steroidal Anti-Inflammatory Drugs (NSAIDs) & Aspirin during Pregnancy

Over 17 million Americans use non-steroidal anti-inflammatory drugs (NSAIDs) for pain relief. Common NSAIDs include aspirin, ibuprofen (Motrin, Advil, Nuprin), naproxen (Aleve), and ketoprofen. While these drugs are safe and often effective under normal circumstances, pregnant women should avoid taking these drugs unless your doctor prescribes them.

{Fun Fact} Aspirin was the first NSAID on the market and is considered the prototype Non-steroidal Anti-Inflammatory Drug.

Because NSAIDs and aspirin can cross the placenta and enter your baby's blood stream, high doses of these drugs can lead to pregnancy complications, including fetal death (miscarriage and stillbirths), slow growth in the womb, and bleeding abnormalities.

Chronic high-dose use of aspirin in your third trimester may lead to prolonged vaginal bleeding and premature closure of your baby's ductus arteriosus – a blood vessel that connects the two major arteries in your little one's heart. When your baby is in the womb, this important blood vessel redirects blood so it does not fill into the baby's non-functioning lungs. (During pregnancy, your baby does not use its lungs because it gets its oxygen from your placenta).

Studies have also linked short-term use of NSAIDs in late pregnancy to a significant increase risk of premature ductus closure. Premature closure of the ductus arteriosus can lead to fetal death.

> **{Fact}** Within 24 hours of the birth, the baby's ductus arteriosus will close on its own because it is no longer needed. When this blood vessel does not close after birth, your baby is said to have patent ductus arteriosus (PDA) – a very common congenital heart defect. This condition occurs in 2 out of every 1,000 full term births, and 8 in every 1,000 premature births.

Taking aspirin close to your delivery may also increase your anemia, prolong your pregnancy, and lengthen your labor.

Aspirin use during pregnancy can also lead to smaller babies and neonatal bruising (your baby's skin is bruised at the time of delivery, and any light touch may cause bruising).

Experts are mixed on the safety of low-dose aspirin use (60 to 150 mg/day) during pregnancy. It does not appear to be linked to birth defects when used in the first trimester. In the second and third trimesters, low-dose aspirin is used in select high-risk patients to reduce the frequency of pregnancy-induced hypertension and preeclampsia (high blood pressure and protein in your urine).

Low-dose aspirin is also used to prevent miscarriages and improve pregnancy outcomes for women with antiphospholipid antibody syndrome—an autoimmune disorder that causes blood clots, which can result in a number of pregnancy complications.

The benefit of low-dose aspirin in regular women with a history of miscarriage remains controversial.

If taken throughout pregnancy, low-dose aspirin should be stopped after 36 weeks. Ideally, it should be stopped at least 1 week before delivery because there is a slight increase of bleeding during the labor and delivery process.

Aspirin and NSAIDs are not recommended for use in low-risk pregnant women. To manage pain or headaches, you may want to take Tylenol (acetaminophen) instead.

{**Fact**} In women with a history of serious blood clots, the benefit for continuing to take low-dose aspirin during labor and delivery outweighs the risk of bleeding.

NORMAL CHANGES TO EXPECT

Goodbye to Morning Sickness

Say goodbye and good riddance to morning sickness – the pregnancy-related nausea and vomiting that has plagued you for the last 3 months. Most women report a significant decrease in morning sickness by the end of their first trimester.

Your morning sickness symptoms will gradually improve, a little each day, until they completely disappear. You may not even be aware that your morning sickness is gone until you stop to think about it.

With your morning sickness gone, you will have more strength, as you're no longer spending hours upon hours throwing up and feeling nauseated. The smells of food will no longer bother you, and you will be hungry for food again.

Your appetite should increase. Don't be surprised if you start to gain weight and find yourself eating at strange hours of the night. The levels of the hormone progesterone in your pregnant body will make you hungry all the time. Just remember to eat a healthy and balanced diet.

{**Fact**} Only 15 to 20 percent of women experience morning sickness until their third trimester. Around 5 percent of pregnant women will have symptoms until their delivery.

In the rare cases that your morning sickness symptoms become so severe that you cannot keep any food down and you become dehydrated, you may have "hyperemesis gravidarum" or severe morning sickness. Less than 2 percent of pregnant women experience this.

Excessive Salivation

Along with the gum changes that we discussed in Week 10, don't be surprised if you find yourself producing more saliva than usual during pregnancy. Called ptyalism, this excess saliva production is an annoying pregnancy symptom that occurs most often in pregnant women who have morning sickness or hyperemesis gravidarum. Although it starts in the first trimester, it can last throughout the second trimester as well.

Doctors do not know what causes this excessive saliva production, but it may be due to hormonal changes in pregnancy.

Some experts believe that ptyalism may be due to these women's inability to swallow normal amounts of saliva rather than an actual increase in their saliva production.

The average person produces between 1 to 2 quarts of saliva every day, but because you unconsciously swallow your saliva, you don't notice how much saliva you actually produce. Pregnant women with morning sickness may try to avoid swallowing to keep their vomiting at bay, and this may make the saliva build up in their mouth and make their natural saliva production more noticeable.

It is also possible that pregnant women salivate more often to relieve the heartburn that is common in pregnancy. When you have heartburn, your stomach acid irritates your esophagus and causes a burning sensation. Because your saliva contains bicarbonate, swallowing neutralizes the acid in your esophagus.

Whatever the reason for this phenomenon, producing more saliva is annoying. Women with ptyalism often have to carry around a cloth or cup to spit into. When they sleep at night, they often have excessive drool.

> **{Fact}** If you have excessive saliva, avoid sour gum and candy, as these will make you produce even more saliva.

COMPLICATIONS DURING PREGNANCY

Measles ("Red Measles")

Measles is a common childhood disease that affects over 10 million people worldwide and kills close to 200,000 people every year. Because of the MMR (measles-mumps-rubella) vaccine, it rarely affects people in the United States. In other parts of the world, however, measles are the leading cause of vaccine-preventable deaths in young children. Also called rubeola or red measles, the measles can affect anyone who has not been vaccinated or had the disease.

Catching the measles during pregnancy can increase your risk for serious complications, including miscarriage, premature birth, and a low birth weight baby. You also face an increased risk of pneumonia.

If you get the measles late in pregnancy, you can pass the virus to your baby. Your baby may develop a rash within 10 days of birth.

> **{Fact}** Do not confuse the measles with the German measles (caused by the rubella virus). The red measles is caused by a different virus, and it lasts for a longer period of time. It does not have as devastating of an impact on your growing baby as the German measles.

The measles is very contagious and it is spread through contact with an infected person. When the sick person sneezes or coughs, he or she spreads the virus into the air. You can be contagious with the virus 4 days before the onset of symptoms and 4 days after the symptoms first appear.

> **{Fact}** Measles is so contagious that 90 percent of the people (who are not immune or vaccinated) around the infected person will catch the virus.

Symptoms of the measles include fever, runny nose and watery eyes, tiny white spots on the lining of your mouth, and a red, blotchy skin rash that begins on your forehead and spreads down your body to your feet.

Measles will go away on its own, so there is no specific treatment for the disease. You may want to take Tylenol (acetaminophen), which is safe to use in pregnancy, to reduce the fever. Your symptoms should go away within 2 weeks.

Once you have had an active measles infection, you will have immunity from the disease for life. Getting a MMR vaccination will also give you immunity.

Because the measles can be harmful during pregnancy, it is important that you have a measles vaccination before pregnancy. You cannot have the MMR vaccination during pregnancy because it contains a live weakened virus.

{Fact} Before the MMR vaccine, almost all children were infected with measles by age 15. Now there are only about 50 cases in the U.S. every year.

Rubella (German Measles)
Similar to the red measles, rubella (also called German measles) is a contagious viral disease that can cause fever and a red rash. It is passed from person to person through droplets from the infected person's nose and throat – i.e. through coughing and sneezing. Unlike the measles, German measles are caused by the rubella virus, and the illness only lasts about 3 days.

The illness tends to be mild in children and non-pregnant adults. Symptoms include a slight fever, a red rash, swollen lymph nodes, and joint pain and swelling. In pregnant women, German measles can create devastating effects in the developing baby.

If you are infected with rubella for the first time during pregnancy, it can pass through the placenta to infect your baby. The German measles can increase your risk of miscarriage, fetal death, birth defects, and preterm baby. The virus causes more harm early in your pregnancy.

If the virus is transmitted to your baby within the first 16 weeks of your pregnancy, your baby has a high risk of developing congenital rubella syndrome (CRS) – a birth defect that can cause mental retardation, deafness, cataracts, heart defects, liver and spleen problems, and bone disease in affected infants.

{Fact} If you contract German measles in the first trimester, your risk of delivering a baby with CRS is 90 percent.

Contracting rubella in the first trimester will cause your baby's CRS symptoms to be more severe, as this is a vital time for fetal organ development. Although your baby can still develop CRS with an infection later in the pregnancy, the risk is low and the symptoms are much milder.

Not all the babies with CRS will show signs at birth. Up to 40 percent of CRS affected babies go on to develop diabetes later in life.

{Fact} Since 2001, only 5 babies in the United States have been born with congenital rubella syndrome (CRS).

Similar to the measles, rubella will resolve on its own. It cannot be treated with antibiotics, as these are not affective against viral infections. Most obstetricians will screen you for antibodies to rubella on your first prenatal visit.

There are no treatment options for pregnant women with rubella, so prevention is key to eliminating CRS. It is important to receive your MMR vaccine before you ever become pregnant.

{Fact} If you had the German measles immediately before your pregnancy, this will not increase your baby's risk of CRS.

Mumps

Another contagious viral disease, mumps is a disease that primarily affects the salivary glands. Like the measles and German measles, it is spread through close contact with sick people. It is considered a childhood disease, but it can affect adults who have not been vaccinated or exposed to the virus.

Although the symptoms of the mumps are mild, it can complicate pregnancy. If you contract the illness in your first trimester, your risk of miscarriage and preterm birth increases. Unlike the German measles, it is not linked with any birth defects.

Similar to the two types of measles, people with the mumps can be contagious even before they develop any symptoms. One in five people with the mumps have no signs of disease. When signs and symptoms do appear, two or three weeks may have passed after exposure to the virus. Symptoms may include fever, weakness, fatigue, pain when you chew and swallow, and swollen and painful salivary glands.

{**Fun Fact**} The swollen salivary glands that come with the mumps can make your cheeks puff out. The term "mumps" is an old expression for describing the "chipmunk cheeks" that you get with this illness.

With no treatment options available, it is important for you to receive the MMR vaccine to prevent this illness before your pregnancy.

{**Fact**} Before the MMR vaccine was introduced in the United States in the 1960s, mumps was a common childhood illness, affecting over 200,000 people. Now the disease is virtually eliminated, though outbreaks still occur in the U.S.

CLOSING REMARKS

Congratulations on completing the first trimester of your pregnancy! As you've read in this book, the second trimester is often called the "honeymoon" period of pregnancy. Many of your pregnancy aches and pains will begin to disappear and fade away, and you will have more energy for everyday life.

In the second trimester, your body and baby will start growing very rapidly. You will look very pregnant within a few weeks. By the beginning of your third trimester, your little one will have formed all of his or her major organs and he or she may be as long as 15 inches and weigh between 2 or 3 pounds! Your baby can also hear your voice for the first time during the second trimester.

The most exciting thing about this part of pregnancy is that you can start to feel your baby move inside your tummy between 17 and 20 weeks. At first, it may feel like a gas bubble or fluttering inside you. As your pregnancy continues, your baby's movement will become much more prominent.

Though you will be feeling better, you should understand that your second trimester does come with different concerns and considerations.

Because your baby is growing so rapidly, stretch marks may begin, even though you won't be able to notice them immediately. Your moles may become larger, and even warts on your skin will be bigger. Some women experience vivid dreams in the middle part of pregnancy. Other unpleasant side effects may include varicose veins, hair and nail changes, changes in your balance, wild mood swings, clumsiness, and forgetfulness.

If you enjoyed this book, check out the next book in this series: *Your Pregnancy MD: The Second Trimester*. Learn about everything you need to know about the middle part of pregnancy, including all the changes you should expect in your baby, your own pregnancy symptoms, changes to expect, complications that may arise, and more!

In *Your Pregnancy MD: The Second Trimester*, there is a bonus Labor and Delivery section to get you prepped and ready for your baby's entry into this world.

Have a Wonderful Rest of this Journey!

AUTHOR'S BIO

Dr. James W. Brann, M.D., FACOG is a retired obstetrician and gynecologist with over 26 years of clinical experience. A graduate of the University of California at Santa Barbara, he continued his education at the University Autonoma de Guadalajara Medical School. He spent one year researching the pharmacokinetics of antibiotics use in pregnancy at the University of California at Irvine. Afterwards, he had two internships, one in pediatrics at Loma Linda University Medical School, and the second in obstetrics and gynecology at the University of Nevada Medical School. His residency was also at the University of Nevada Medical School. He worked in private practice from 1986 until his retirement. He is author of "Surviving the Joy of Pregnancy" (Xlibris, 2007) and is president and editorial director of Women's Healthcare Topics (www.womenshealthcaretopics.com), a Web site devoted to educating women on healthcare issues.

{Index}

A

Birth weight *(continued)*

    decongestant use in first trimester, 132

    gum disease linked to, 96

    heroin and narcotics use and risk of, 43

    inflammatory bowel disease (IBD) risk for, 97

    measles infection during pregnancy and, 142

    pneumonia during pregnancy and, 109

    urinary tract infections and, 36

Bladder infections, 66

    See also Infections

Bleeding

    implantation, 7, 10-11, 16, 50, 63

    vaginal

        after delivery, 78

        after sexual intercourse, 11, 65, 117

        amniocentesis complication, 93

        aspirin use and, 139

        cervical polyp and, 64

        cocaine (drug) use and, 43

        ectopic pregnancy and, 12-13

        genital warts and, 64

        in early pregnancy, 7, 62-63

        placenta previa and, 104

        signs of miscarriage, 46, 63

        signs of molar pregnancy, 16, 23

        smoking and risk of, 9, 41

        swollen labia and, 64

        uterine fibroid and, 64-65

        vaginal infections and, 64

        vanishing twin and, 49, 64

Bloating, 8, 9, 18, 44-45, 69

Body mass index (BMI), 28-29

Bradley method, 15

Breast

    changes in pregnancy, 10, 27, 94-95

    engorged, 62

    leaking (colostrum), 95

    Montgomery's tubercles, 27, 95, 114

    nipple changes, 27, 94

    sensitivity, 8, 27, 94

    stretch marks, 95

    swollen, 10, 27, 94

    tenderness, 8, 10, 94

    See also Maternity bras

Breastfeeding

    as birth control, 105

    HIV infection and, 62

    infection passed through, 62, 123

    inverted nipples and, 95

    irritable bowel disease (IBD) and, 98

    safety of HPV vaccine while, 78

C

Caffeine

    miscarriage risk, 24, 31, 47

    frequent urination, 46

Caladryl lotion (Praxoxine), 137

Calamine lotion, 137

Calcium, 20, 53, 54, 55, 56, 99

Carrier test, 91

    See also Anemia and Birth defects

Cervical polyps, 50, 63, 64

Cesarean delivery (c-sections), 14, 29, 58, 62

Chloasma, 114

Choriocarcinoma, 78-79

    See also Gestational trophoblastic disease (GTD) and Molar

Mylanta, 135

N

Naproxen (Aleve), 138

Narcotic (drug), harmful effects of, 43

Nasal congestion, 118-120
    medication to treat, 131, 133

Nasal sprays, 120, 131

Nausea and vomiting. *See* Morning sickness

Neosporin (ointment), 135

Neural tube defects
    folic acid and prevention of, 20, 55, 90
    screening for, 91, 92, 93
    spina bifida, 89

Non-steroidal anti-inflammatory drugs (NSAIDs), 138-140

Nosebleeds, 118-120

Nuchal translucency screening, 92
    See also Ultrasound

Nutrition. *See* Diet

O

Oatmeal bath, 137

Obesity, 70, 90

Orgasm, 116

Osteoporosis, 56, 89

Ovarian cysts, 118

Ovulation, 2, 56, 70, 105

P

Pap smear, 66, 77
    abnormal, 67, 77-78

PCP (drug), harmful effects of, 43-44

Pelvis
    lightning, 45-46
    pelvic exam, 63, 66

pelvic inflammatory disease, 12, 13

pelvic pressure and pain, 23, 106-107

uterus rises above, 113

Pica, 58

Placenta
    abruption. *See* Placental abruption
    attachment to uterus and impact of smoking, 41
    blood clots developing in, 48
    development, 6, 17, 106
    diagnostic testing and, 93
    drugs and medicine crossing the, 42, 130-131, 138
    fetal protection, 107
    high blood pressure and, 57
    infection through, 60, 109, 143
    in molar pregnancy, 23
    in choriocarcinoma, 78
    previa. *See* Placenta Previa

Placenta previa, 41, 104, 117

Placental abruption, 41, 43, 104

Pneumonia, 109, 142

Polysporin (ointment), 135

Preeclampsia, 132, 139
    See also High blood pressure

Premature birth
    alcohol use and risk of, 40
    anemia and risk of, 98
    back-to-back pregnancy and risk of, 105
    blood clots and, 48
    definition of, 3
    drug abuse and risk of, 9, 42, 44
    German measles (rubella), 143
    flu and risk of, 109, 111

Unbilical cord *(continued)*
    in diagnostic testing, 94
Unisom (doxylamine), 136
Unplanned pregnancy
    choices in, 71-75
    shock of, 67
    while on birth control pill, 70-71
Urination, frequency of, 7, 8, 18-19,
    45-46
Urinary tract infections (UTI), 35-36
Uterus
    abortion, risk of damage to, 75
    choriocarcinoma development, 78
    endometriosis and, 13, 56
    ectopic pregnancy and, 41
    growth of, 19, 45, 52, 59, 69, 102,
        106, 107, 113, 114, 117, 118,
        125, 128-129
    implantation in, 6, 7, 16, 63
    lining of, 70
    placenta attachment, 41, 93
    molar pregnancy development,
      22
    shape of uterus, 47
    uterine fibroids and, 64-65
    weight of, 21, 45, 46, 52, 53, 69

V

Vaginal bleeding. *See* Bleeding
Vaginal infections. *See* Infections
Vanishing twin syndrome, 48-49, 63,
    64
    See also Miscarriage
Vegetarian and vegan diets, 39, 50,
    54-56
    See also Diet
Vena cava vein, 21
Vicks Cough Syrup, 133

Vitamin A, 55
    See also Diet
Vitamin B12, 56
    See also Diet
Vitamin B6 (pyridoxine), 34, 136
    See also Diet
Vitamin C, 55, 99
    See also Diet
Vitamin D, 54, 55
    See also Diet
Vomiting. *See* Morning Sickness

W

Waistline expansion, 106-107
Weight gain. *See* Diet
Witch hazel, 136

X

X-Linked Disorder, 85-86
    See also Birth defects and Genetic
      disorder
X-rays. *See* Radiation

Y

Yeast infection, 64, 137-138
Yolk sac, 6, 17, 18

Z

Zantac, 135